YOGIC CURE FOR COMMON AILMENTS

How to use yoga exercises in the treatment of illness.

YOGIC CURE FOR COMMON AILMENTS

The therapeutic application of Yoga

Phulgenda Sinha

THORSONS PUBLISHERS LIMITED
Wellingborough, Northamptonshire

© Dr Phulgenda Sinha 1980

Published in arrangement with
Vision Books Private Limited,
36C Connaught Place, New Delhi 1100 001, India.

This revised edition for UK and
Western Markets 1980

© THORSONS PUBLISHERS LIMITED 1980

British Library Cataloguing in Publication Data

Sinha, Phulgenda
    Yogic cure for common ailments. - Revised
ed.
    1. Yoga - Therapeutic use
    I. Title
    615'.89   RM727.Y64

ISBN 0-7225-0590-6

Typeset by Elanders Computer Assisted
Typesetting Systems
and printed and bound in Great Britain by
Cox & Wyman Ltd, Reading

Contents

To my wife Shanti Devi

Publisher's Note

This book is a reference work based on the research and practical experience of the author, and whilst they have been written in good faith the directions given in this book should not be considered as a substitute for consultation with a qualified doctor.

Preface

This book is the product of my years of experience in treating patients of various diseases, disorders and ailments through yoga. My experience at the Yoga Institute in Washington D.C.,U.S.A. from 1965 to 1968 and at the Indian Institute of Yoga, Patna since 1969 has inspired me to write on therapeutic yoga.

Everything written, every *asana* prescribed, and every advice given in this book is based on my research and personal experience during the treatment of patients, and readers will have no difficulty in treating themselves by following the guidelines given. There is no need to disrupt the routine of normal life while practising the prescribed yoga *asanas*. The diet in every case is almost normal. Though the diet chart is provided separately for every disease, the general principles and methods of eating remain the same as recommended to any practiser of yoga.

The *asanas*, *pranayamas* and other *kriyas* recommended for treating a particular disease are such and so illustrated that a person of any physique would be able to practise them easily. In case of some difficult *asanas*, their easier forms have been explained and illustrated together with the original ones.

It is very disheartening to note that a great majority of the books on therapeutic yoga make it compulsory for the patients to do the *kriyas* of *Shat Karmas* (the six purificatory processes) as a prerequisite for practising yoga for therapeutic purposes. It is true that most of the early books on yoga, such as, *Gherand Samhita, Goraksha Paddhati, Hatha Pradipika* and *Vasistha Samhita* speak very highly about the benefits of these *Shat Karmas* and provide the details of practising them. But it should be remembered that these *Shat Karmas* were primarily recommended for a few chosen *Sadhakas* (disciples) whose training in the yoga system was mainly for achieving spiritual, religious and devotional ends.

It should also be remembered that the *Sadhakas* who were asked to perform the *Shat Karmas* were already in good health and they practised these techniques with a notion of purifying themselves for gaining the divine powers rather than getting cured of diseases. Since most of the teachers of yoga therapy today still recommend their practises to the patients and also to the general public; let me enumerate these *Shat Karmas* and explain why they are not recommended to the users of this book.

The *Shat Karmas* are the six purificatory

techniques or processes. They are: *Dhauti, Basti, Neti, Trataka, Nauli* and *Kapalbhati*. One major reason for not recommending these purificatory processes is that unless done properly, they might cause grave injury and severe damage to those practising them. Those who are interested in learning any or all of these purificatory techniques must do so in the presence of the teacher and not with the help of any book, no matter how comprehensively written. This book is written as a guide for self-treatment and thus it should be obvious that the practise of these purificatory processes cannot be advised.

In selecting the topics of this book I have been faced with a problem–what to include and what to exclude. There are several diseases and ailments which I had the opportunity to treat, such as tuberculosis, parkinsonism, ulcer, polio, leucorrhoea, impotency, etc., but they have not been covered in this book. One major reason for excluding them has been that the number of patients treated for these diseases was not enough to justify the claim of curing through therapeutic yoga as a proven system of treatment. And secondly, the size of the book.

I have decided to cover only those diseases and disorders which are very common and of which I have long experience of treating numerous patients. With these considerations, I have covered *(i)* Abdominal Disorders, *(ii)* Diabetes, *(iii)* Asthma, *(iv)* Arthritis, *(v)* Obesity, *(vi)* Mental Problems and *(vii)* Heart ailments and

High Blood Pressure, in this book.

The first chapter which is an introductory chapter, explains the value, method and essentials of therapeutic yoga and it provides a guideline for making use of a particular chapter for the treatment of a particular disease.

For general practisers of yoga also this will be a useful book. The method of practising *asanas, pranayamas* and other *kriyas* are clearly explained step by step along with the illustrations so that even beginners will have no difficulty in following them with accuracy. By selecting *asanas* according to the suitability of body conditions any person can learn yoga with the help of this book.

1.

Therapeutic Yoga and its Essentials

Therapeutic yoga is basically a system of self-treatment. According to the yogic view, diseases, disorders and ailments are the result of faulty ways of living, bad habits, and improper food. The diseases are thus the resultant state of a short or prolonged malfunctioning of the body system.

Since the root cause of most diseases lies in the mistakes of the individual, its cure also lies in correcting those mistakes by the same individual. Thus, it is the individual himself who is held responsible in both the cases, that is, for causing as well as for curing the disease. The yoga expert shows only the path and works no more than as a counsellor to the patient.

The yogic treatment of disease comprises diet, yoga practice, and correct thinking and natural living.

Diet

The diet is recommended according to the nature of the disease and the condition of the patient. The main idea about diet is to keep it balanced and at the same time eliminate those items from the daily intake which are considered harmful. A diet-chart for breakfast, lunch, tea, and dinner is prepared for each patient according to his physical condition and the nature of his disease

The most common items of diet permitted for almost all patients of therapeutic yoga are fruits, salad, leafy vegetables, green vegetables, wheat bread and pulses(selected). For the non-vegetarians, fish and liver are allowed in certain cases but meat is generally forbidden. Whatever are the variations in the diet-chart of patients, they are all asked to follow some basic principles of eating which are: to eat slowly, not to eat to their full capacity, to eat at least two hours before going to bed, to avoid drinking water while eating, not to eat hot, spicy, fried and roasted food, not to take more than one or two cups of coffee or tea a day(if possible, cut it out altogether), to give up the use of tobacco in any form, and to avoid the use of alcohol.

Yoga Practice

The patient is asked to practise yoga according to his disease and his bodily condition. In the majority of cases, a regular practice of only a few *asanas* is enough for treating the disease. In some of the diseases the practice of *pranayama* together with the *asanas* becomes essential for good results. In certain cases, specific *kriyas* such as *bandhas, mudras* and certain yogic techniques are used for the desired result. Besides these, the practice of concentration and meditation is also necessary in certain cases.

In our research at the Indian Institute of Yoga Patna, we have found that a large number of illnesses are alleviated within two months of Yoga practice. In certain cases, it takes about four months or even more.

It is interesting to note that the same *asanas, pranayamas, bandhas, mudras* and other *kriyas* which are practised for creative, preventive and general health purposes, are practised also for treating diseases. But there is a difference in the manner of practice by a patient and that of the general student. The patient of a particular disease is advised to practise only as much of an *asana* as is possible for him.

By doing only what is physically performable, the patient gains in strength as the *kriyas* begin to condition the body and diminish the disease. When the sufferer recovers from the illness, physical ability improves and the same *asanas* are performed better even by those who were unable to do them at the beginning.

The yoga therapy is a specialized form of

yogic culture and various yoga centres in India have developed their own systems on the basis of their experience and research. In the absence of any standardization, there is some variation in the method of therapeutic yoga at various centres in India and elsewhere.

Lifestyle
Though most of the patients are cured with proper diet and yoga practice, there are some cases which are rather complicated. Some patients develop diseases and disorders on account of their unhealthy habits and lack of proper knowledge about life, nature and society.

In such cases, a lot of things need to be told to the patient which are informative, conceptual, theoretical and also philosophical. It is time-consuming work. Yogic literature is very rich in this respect and is divided into two main categories: (i) spiritual interpretation of things, and (ii) scientific interpretation of things. However, the literature available in the second category is much less than that in the first one. The readers are best advised to take a scientific approach in all their reading on yoga. Depending upon the nature of disease, a patient is counselled and informed in detail about the various relevant aspects of life.

Following this short description of the method of therapeutic yoga, I will now explain how it differs from orthodox systems of treatment.

Yoga Versus Orthodox System

In any medical system the primary reliance is on medicine. It is assumed that a particular medicine will cure a particular disease. The medical doctor does the diagnosis, identifies the disease and prescribes a suitable medicine. The patient in this system has to do very little or nothing at all. The task of correcting the disease and disorder and restoring the health is assigned to the medicine.

Seen in this context, there is a contrast between the medical system and yoga system of treatment. Whereas in the medical system an external agent (medicine) does the corrective work, in the yoga system this external agent is not needed at all. As said earlier, it is the patient himself whose personal understanding, practice and care alleviates his disease.

It would not be improper to mention that we encountered several patients suffering from various chronic diseases, who had lost their faith in the medical system because in spite of years of treatment they had not achieved a permanent and satisfactory cure. In certain cases, the medicine provided them with immediate relief, but not a lasting cure. On the other hand, a great number of such patients achieved permanent help through therapeutic yoga within a period of two to four months. This has specially been so in cases of diabetes, arthritis, asthma, gastro-intestinal disorders, nervous tension and various other cases.

This limitation of the medical system does not mean that it is inferior to the yoga system; there are areas where only medical science and not yoga can come to the rescue of the patient. Similarly, there are certain diseases, which, though regarded incurable through a medical system, are definitely alleviated through yoga. This shows that every system of treatment has certain unique points as well as limitations.

Therefore, it would be prudent on the part of the medical men to adopt and use this tested ancient system of yoga for treating those diseases and ailments whose medicinal cure is not certain. Since the system of therapeutic yoga is now scientifically established, it can be used as a 'self-cure method' by people suffering from various disorders in any part of the world. Let me now explain its essentials which one must know for making proper use of therapeutic yoga.

Essentials of Yoga Practice
People about to use this book as a guide for self-treatment through yoga need first to be told about the suitability of time, place, physical condition, dress and similar other matters. In order to derive the full benefit from therapeutic yoga it is necessary to understand the following requirements and principles related to its practices.

Time: Though the morning time, before breakfast, is regarded as best for practising yoga, one can do it also in the evening or at any other time, provided the stomach is empty and not heavy with food. The main thing to remember is wait for three or four hours after eating before practising yoga. Also a gap of half an hour or so should be given after drinking water, tea or any juice. The body should be in a restful and normal condition at the time.

The individual should select a time which is convenient for his daily routine and should *try to do yoga at the same time every day.* A practice for at least five to six days in a week should be enough to show improvement. The patients are advised to practise yoga only once in twenty-four hours unless specifically told to do so more often than that.

Place: Practise yoga on the floor. Avoid using a bed. Use a carpet, rug, blanket or mat on the floor. The place of practice should be neat, clean and well ventilated. There should be a constant supply of fresh air. Windows should be kept open for cross-ventilation. During summer, a fan can be used, but during winter take care to avoid cold draughts.

Silence: One should maintain silence while doing yoga. Any conversation, mental activity, and even listening to music should be avoided. Silence helps in preserving energy as well as in being attentive during practice.

Rest: There are two types of rest in yoga: the short rest and the long rest. The short rest should be for about six to eight seconds only. This is taken in between two rounds of the *asanas* or between one and the other *asana.* The shorter rest is completed by breathing twice at the completion of one round of a posture.

The long rest comes at the end of all the *asanas, pranayamas* and other *kriyas* which one does at a stretch. The general principle is to devote a quarter of the actual practising time for this rest. For example, if one has done yoga for twenty minutes, the rest at the end should be for five minutes.

This rest is better done in the position of *Shava asana* (*Savasana*). Those who cannot do *Shava asana* should just lie down on the floor, keeping the eyes closed, body relaxed, breathing normal, and concentrating the mind on any place of natural beauty such as a garden, park or hillside. In this simple method of resting there should be a feeling as if one is breathing the air of that chosen place and is relaxing by being mentally present there. After the rest is over, one should wait for three to five minutes before eating or doing any other routine work.

Dress: The minimium amount of clothes should be worn while practising. In winter, light, woollen clothes can be worn provided they do not restrict movement in any way.

Bath: People generally want to know whether a bath should be taken before or after yoga practice. For those practising yoga in the morning, it is not necessary to take a bath before they do it. It depends on convenience and personal choice whether to bathe before or after the practice. When taking a hot bath after yoga practice one must wait for about fifteen minutes. Many people prefer to practice yoga after taking a bath because there are certain *asanas* which are done better after a bath and it creates a feeling of neatness and purity.

Method of practice: In order to obtain the fullest benefit from yoga, one must practise it in the proper way. Since yoga is a scientific system it requires to be done in a specified manner. If the *asanas, pranayamas, bandhas* and *mudras* are not done according to the established methods, it will become merely an exercise and will not give satisfactory results.

What is more important here to mention is that though not everyone can practice all the postures with perfection, they can certainly follow the method of doing them without any difficulty. Therefore the advice is: do yoga according to the limits of your body. Do it only as much as you can. You need not be perfect in forms. If you cannot do the full form, do half of it or even less.

Follow all the steps carefully. Another important piece of advice is to begin the practice with only a few *asanas* during the first week. When two or three *asanas* have been practised for a week, the next two *asanas* should be added during the second week. This way every week new *asanas* can be added gradually according to the need and recommendation in a given case.

Female problems: Women should avoid yoga practice during a menstrual period and during advanced stage (after the fourth month) of pregnancy. Under such conditions yoga practice should be generally discontinued. Yoga for pregnant women (after the fourth month) has to be performed on a selective basis under the proper care and instructions of a yoga expert.

It is significant to mention that yoga has great value for eliminating various feminine ailments and disorders. It also works as an aid to their health. For example, menstrual disorders can be corrected and normalized through yoga. Proper practice of yoga during the early stages of pregnancy enhances the health of the child in the womb and it also helps to make the delivery painless.

How Much Yoga? Yoga can be practised for a longer time in the winter season than in summer. Maximum time devoted to actually practising yoga should not exceed forty-five minutes in a single day of winter. In summer, the maximum time for actual practice should be thirty minutes. Time for rest may be allowed in addition according to the principle mentioned above. This difference in practising time has to be maintained because of the variation in the effect of weather on the body.

Though there should be only one session of yoga practice a day, those who would like to divide their time in two sessions should allow a gap of eight hours between the first and the second session. A minimum practice of fifteen minutes per day should be quite satisfactory for maintaining good health.

With the above-mentioned clarifications about therapeutic yoga and its basic requirements, I will now explain what is meant by 'proper diet' in the yoga system. A proper understanding of the established principles and advice about diet would help people to realize the importance of food and its effect on the body in a better way. Though specific diet-charts are already mentioned for different types of diseases, the users of this book are advised to read the following section on diet for a comprehensive knowledge of it.

A Balanced Diet

Diet occupies a dominant place in the yoga system. It is said that 'you are what you eat'. This is because the kind and quality of food affects the physical as well as mental condition of the individual. Thus, the individual who does not take a proper diet and who does not have a proper understanding of the principles of eating, gradually begins to harm himself both physically and mentally. He begins to feel the ill-effects of wrong eating habits on his appearance, behaviour, thought and action.

In yoga, all foods have been divided into three categories: *Rajasi, Tamasi* and *Sattvik.* These are explained below.

Rajasi: The *rajasi* food comprises a variety of dishes. It derives its name from the eating habits of Indian kings. It is said that no less than fifty-six dishes were served at a royal dining table. Naturally, in these types of preparations, dishes of various kinds – some fried, some roasted, and some curried and highly seasoned – together with various sweets and drinks would be served. Foods of this type are regarded as undesirable for the yoga student as they create extra weight and fat, generate a feeling of heaviness for a longer period of time after dinner, and arouse passion.

Tamasi: The second category is *tamasi* which includes foods which are prepared hot. When any dish – vegetarian or non-vegetarian – is prepared with too many spices and with excessive use of salt, pepper, chilli and similar other seasonings, it becomes *tamasi.* This type of food suits those who have a coarse nature and a rough temperament, and are inclined to be noisy, quarrelsome and intolerant. Hence, this type of food is undesirable and not recommended to the followers of yoga.

Sattvik: In this type, the food is cooked with the least amount of spices and without much seasoning. Though the food is fresh, attractive and nutritive, it is cooked in a simple way. This type of food is desirable and highly recommended for those practising yoga.

According to yogic principles no food, whether vegetarian or non-vegetarian, is by itself *rajasi, tamasi* or *sattvik.* What makes it this or that type is the method of preparation and not the food by itself. The generally held notion that the non-vegetarian food is *tamasi* and the vegetarian food is *sattvik*, is wrong, because potato or cauliflower can be prepared as *tamasi* and meat or chicken can be cooked as *sattvik*, depending upon the choice of the individual.

The second point which needs clarification is that, in yoga, foods are not evaluated on the basis of their calorific count. Rather it is the quality of the food and the method of eating that are considered. The better the quality of food, the more invigorating it is considered. Many people attempt to lose weight by reducing their intake of food or reducing the calories. Similarly, many people feel that by eating heavily, they could gain weight. These weight control methods are undesirable, as both these extremes have a harmful effect on the individual. Whether a person is overweight or underweight, the yogic principles and methods of eating remain the same. One can gain or lose weight without any ill-effects on his health by following the yogic method of eating. What are then the yogic principles of eating?

Yoga Diet
The most important principle is to eat a balanced diet. When the following four things are included in everyday diet, the diet should become more balanced. These items are: salad, fresh vegetables, fresh fruits and raw nuts. Whether you are a vegetarian or non-vegetarian, you should include these four items with your major dishes of the day.

Salad: All the vegetables that are eaten raw, constitute salad. Things such as cucumber, tomato, carrots, lettuce, cauliflower, etc., can be used for preparing salad. These should be cut into pieces and with a little dressing, can be eaten raw in the quantity of about a cupful per day. The ideal time to eat salad is to make it as the first item of lunch and dinner.

Fresh vegetables: Any vegetables which are not dried or processed in any way, can be regarded as fresh. They are to be preferred as fresh as possible. Fresh vegetables whether from under or above the ground, must be eaten every day. They should, of course, be prepared in a *sattvik* way.

Fresh fruits: Fruits constitute the most nutritive food for any individual. For better results from yogic practice, fresh fruits are essential. It is not necessary to eat only expensive fruits, but any fruits that are easily available would serve the purpose. These fruits can be taken singly or mixed with various types. They can be seasonal or year-round available types. One apple, one orange, and one banana a day, for example, would be enough for an individual. The important point is that fruits should be eaten regularly for better health.

Raw nuts: Those nuts which are taken from hard shells such as cashew, pistachio, almond, pecan and walnuts are recommended. A handful of a mixture of these nuts would be sufficient for a day. Since these raw nuts have a warm effect on the body, they should be taken in the winter and should be avoided or taken less in summer. Nuts from hard shells are full of protein, minerals, and vitamins. Therefore, a proper intake of these nuts is very energizing and healthy for the practisers and non–practisers of yoga alike.

Besides the above-mentioned items of balanced diet, there are some other principles of diet which must be followed for a satisfactory result. They are as follows.

Quantity of Food

Do not over-eat and don't even eat to your full capacity. When food intake is kept below one's full capacity, it is easily digested and the body makes fuller use of the intake. On the other hand, when food is taken excessively and the stomach is completely full, it is not properly digested and the body is forced to eliminate it without making proper use of it. Further, by eating more the individual is overstraining the abdominal system in particular and the body in general, and the performances of his physical and mental powers are obstructed. Putting on extra and unnecessary weight is the natural outcome of overeating.

Method of Eating

The proper method is to eat slowly and swallow the food after thoroughly crushing and chewing it. One common error which overweight people generally make is that they eat too fast. It appears that fast-eaters develop a habit wherein they derive satisfaction from food only when they gulp it.

The yogic system, thus takes into consideration the ill-effects of fast eating and emphasizes the importance of slow eating. But the question is: How slow? It depends on the type of food one is eating. For example, a banana can be chewed faster than an apple. Meat eating would take more time than fish. But in all circumstances, the guideline is to chew the food thoroughly and only then should it be swallowed. There are many benefits of slow eating. The individual gets full satisfaction from his food even when he eats only a small quantity. Saliva can be properly mixed up with the food and make it easily digestible. The body makes full use of any food taken and the individual maintains better health by a smaller amount of food.

Time Factor: Eat at least two hours before going to bed. A common error with most people is that they eat and then soon go to sleep, especially during the night time. This has a very harmful effect upon their health. By eating well before going to bed the food is properly processed by the body. The stomach is not heavy and when the individual goes to sleep, he gets undisturbed sleep and rest. Most people, who complain of abdominal, stomach or bowel troubles, are in the habit of eating and then immediately going to sleep. By so doing, they put undue strain on the abdominal muscles.

They get disturbed sleep and most of the time they suffer from digestion ailments and disorders.

Another important aspect which needs clarification is how many times a day one should eat. It is recommended that one should eat four times within a period of twenty-four hours. This means having breakfast in the morning, lunch at noon, some refreshment in the afternoon and dinner in the evening. It is up to the individual to eat according to his choice and preference, while keeping in mind the yogic principles. Unless one is faced with some special occasion, eating four times a day should be made a habit of daily life.

Spices: It is recommended not to use too many spices while preparing various dishes. This means not too much salt, chilli, peppers and other herbs. That is not to say that spices are bad. The objection is to excessive use of spices and seasoning. The seasoning can be done for flavour, but excessive use should be avoided. The food should be so seasoned that it does not become *tamasi*, but remains *sattvik* in nature.

Water: It is recommended that the practisers of yoga should drink about five pints (about ten to twelve glasses) of water every day. Water should not be taken at the time of eating, but after half-an-hour of eating. According to yogic literature, several skin diseases and disorders can be corrected if water is not taken while eating. The drinking of plenty of water is highly recommended in yogic literature, because it is held that water cleans and washes out the impurities of the system. Many people do not drink enough water.

I have known some people who were in the habit of drinking little or no water at all. Instead of water, they used to take juice, milk and other liquids. As a result, they developed a number of ailments and physical disorders. But most of these ailments were corrected when they started taking plenty of water every day.

Coffee and Tea: Both coffee and tea are injurious to health when taken in excess. Modern people are now so used to tea and coffee in their daily lives that it is not easy to give them up. But a restraint on their intake must be maintained for better health. It is recommended that not more than two cups of tea or coffee should be taken in a period of twenty-four hours. There are various reasons for this. Both these drinks, if taken in large quantities, cause constipation, insomnia, nervous tension and internal disorders. It has also been felt that an excess intake of these beverages distorts the natural complexion of the skin and produces a roughening effect on the facial tissues.

Alcoholic Drinks: All alcoholic drinks are regarded as vitamin thieves. They steal and destroy the nutrients of the system. The objection to taking alcoholic drinks is not because they are intoxicating but mainly because they weaken the individual, physically and mentally, if taken without restraint. Regardless of high or low alcoholic percentage in a drink, if a daily habit of drinking is maintained, it would prove extremely harmful. Therefore it is advisable to avoid making the habit of taking these drinks every day.

Gram (chickpeas): Sprouted gram (chickpeas) is a very nutritious food. It is full of protein, minerals and vitamins. A regular intake of a handful of germinated gram is highly conducive to good health. Practisers of yoga are, therefore, advised to make it a part of their daily eating. Green grams can be eaten fresh. The ripe ones should be eaten after soaking in water for about eight hours. The sprouted grams are better than the plain ones, as the sprouted ones are enriched with energy derived from the air and light. If a person is not able to eat raw nuts and fruits regularly, he can compensate this loss by eating sprouted grams regularly.

The recommendations on diet can be summed up by saying that yogic principles of diet are so simple that the yoga practisers (whether vegetarian or non-vegetarian) should have no difficulty in following them. If these principles are followed closely and if the individual makes a habit of eating according to these recommendations, he will maintain good health. A good balanced diet along with proper hygienic care, and regular yoga practice will ensure good health.

Hygiene
Since enough has been said about proper diet and other requirements for the yoga practitioners, I shall explain what is meant by hygienic care.

Bathing and Washing: Water is one of the three important things for the survival of human beings. The other important items are air and food. We know that several plants flourish on water and that some people can survive on water alone for several weeks and even months. This shows that in water there are life nourishing elements. This being the importance of water, the followers of yoga must make proper use of it by taking sufficient water.

In summer, one can bathe twice daily. In the other seasons, bathing once a day is necessary for maintaining good health. One can use hot or cold water for bathing according to personal liking and the weather.

It also needs to be explained how this external use of water benefits the individual. For this, we have to understand the structural and functional aspects of *romekoops* (pores).

The word *romekoop* is made of two Sanskrit words (*rome koop*). *Rome* means hair and *koop* means well. Thus its literal meaning would be a hair-well, which is called pore in English. We have millions of hairs on our body and the root of each of them goes deeper in the body from the upper layer of the skin. At the root of every hair there is a tiny hole which is not visible to the naked eye. These tiny holes at the roots of

the hairs are called *romekoops*. The body dis-
cards sweat and impurities of the system
through these *romekoops* and allows penetration of air, water, etc., through them. Since
these pores work as passages to and from the
internal cells of the body for perspiration and
absorption, the yogic system makes good use of
them.

Hence, the primary consideration is how to
make good use of the pores in order to benefit
the system. This is achieved by rubbing the
whole body thoroughly while taking a bath, as
it serves several purposes.

Rubbing the Body: There are several ways of
rubbing the body during a bath, such as with the
palms, sponge, flannel or brush. But the best
thing to rub the body with, is a flannel. The
process is to get the flannel soaked in water,
apply some soap to it and rub the whole body
with it briskly while taking a bath. This rubbing
serves several purposes. It opens the pores, and
stimulates the upper layers of the skin. This
rubbing can be done with or without using soap.
After rubbing, plenty of fresh water should be
poured on the body.

Use of Soaps: In our modern times, it is very
difficult to think of bathing without using soap.
Though principles are not opposed to using
soap, it must be understood that there can be
certain chemicals in it which do not suit the skin
type of every individual. Many people get
rashes and rough skin after using certain types

of soaps. Also, except for cleaning the body, soaps do not contribute much to the good of the body. Thus, it is suggested that if you must use soap, select a good quality which is agreeable to your skin.

In the yogic system, the method of cleaning is different. There are several substitutes for soap. These substitutes not only clean the body but also contribute potentially to the health of the body. Amongst the yogic usable things, some are not available everywhere. Therefore, a simple but good material is recommended for this purpose.

One good substitute for soap is gram (chickpea) flour. Take a handful or more of gram flour and make a paste with lukewarm water in a pot. While taking a bath, rub the whole body with this paste. Rub it with the palms. After this rubbing wash it with hot or cold water. The body will be cleaner than with soap and it will become smooth, soft and invigorated with energy. It can also be mentioned that gram flour alleviates many skin diseases and troubles such as itching, rough skin and similar other skin disorders.

It is recommended that it should be used at intervals of two to three days. This flour can also be used for cleaning the face and shampooing hair. For cleaning the face the process remains the same as for cleaning the body, but for shampooing the hair some extra work is involved.

Shampooing: Take the kneaded flour and make

a paste of it. Then put it in some thin cloth and tie it up. Now squeeze the cloth containing the paste in water till the soft part is mixed with water and only the debris remains in the cloth. When it has been well squeezed in water, throw the debris left in the cloth away and use the remaining liquid type paste for shampooing hair. Squeezing the paste is done to filter it in such a way that its large grains are out and they do not get stuck in the hair. The filtered paste will clean the hair in a very satisfactory and healthy way. Those who prefer to use other types of shampoos should choose a really suitable kind for cleaning the hair. Hair should be shampooed once or at most twice a week.

Hair: Hair is the index of health of the individual. Healthy hair generally means a healthy person. One simple way to keep the hair healthy is to rub the roots when taking a bath. The process is to wet the hair and rub with finger-tips at the roots until a warming-up effect is felt. After rubbing for a minute or so, rinse the hair with plenty of water and dry with a clean towel. The hair should be combed thoroughly two or three times daily as this makes it stronger and prevents it from falling.

Some people have a false idea that by rubbing and combing, they would lose their hair. Though someone who has dandruff might lose some hair by rubbing and combing in the initial stage, the falling of their hair would stop after a week or so. New hair would soon begin to grow in any case. This rubbing and combing method is equally good for men and women.

Teeth: Like hair, teeth also symbolize the health of an individual. The simple way of keeping the teeth healthy is to brush them and massage the roots. Besides the morning cleaning, teeth must be brushed before retiring at night.

The brushing should be done in upward and downward motions and not sideways. The next thing is to rub the root of the teeth. This is done by taking some paste on the fingers and putting the thumb inside and the index finger outside and then rubbing the gums firmly. It is sufficient to rub the gums with paste or tooth-powder once a day. This makes the gums grow stronger and stops decay.

Oil Massage: Among various oils used for massaging, mustard oil is the best. Mustard oil is very commonly used in India for cooking, applying to the hair, etc. It is a healthy and invigorating oil. Since it has a warm effect on the body, yoga students are advised to apply it only during the winter not during summer. When it is applied to the body, it penetrates through the pores and imparts elasticity and strength to the muscles, bones and nerves. It soothes, cleans, gives a good, tanned complexion to the body and makes the skin healthy. It also helps to remove wrinkles and dryness of the skin.

Take some oil on the palms and smear it on the body and rub lightly. Apply it all over the body and leave it there for about ten to fifteen minutes during which time, most of the oil will be soaked by the body through the pores.

You can clean the oil from the body in two ways, taking either a bath or a shower without using soap and rub the body using either warm or cold water as preferred. After the bath or shower, remove the surplus oil from the body with a dry, clean towel. As the oil is wiped off, the body will gain a clean and smooth look.

The second process is that after you have applied the oil, apply gram-flour paste as a substitute for soap. Apply the paste all over the body and rub it with the palms till the paste is fully mixed up with the oil that remains on the body. After the rubbing is done, wash it off with either cold or hot water. Gram flour paste will clean the oil in a more thorough and satisfactory way than soap can. By so doing, you have the benefit of both oil and flour. This can be regarded as a beautifying treatment, as it enhances the natural look of the skin.

This application of oil and cleaning with the paste should be done on alternate days, or once or twice a week, but not every day. If you prefer to use soap in between the applications of oil and paste, there is no reason why you shouldn't. In case any soap is used, it should be a kind which is agreeable to the nature and condition of the user's skin type.

Let me sum up this chapter by saying that all the basic information and suggestions in the preceding pages regarding therapeutic yoga have been carefully thought out. You are advised first to read this whole chapter carefully so that you develop a proper understanding of this yogic system of treatment and then start the actual practice. Remember that you are following a system of self-treatment without relying on or using medicine. Therefore, it is important that you understand it from the start for a satisfactory result. Keeping in mind the contents of this chapter, select the section of your concern and begin the practice of yoga according to the guidelines given therein.

2.

Abdominal Disorders

All troubles that disturb the normal functioning of the digestive system have been termed here as abdominal disorders. The commonly found disorders in this case are: constipation, flatulence, indigestion, dysentery, diarrhoea, acidity, stomach ache, and various forms of gastrointestinal disorders. It is a widely prevalent problem of our time affecting young and old alike. Though the causes of abdominal disorders could be varied and multiple, the most common are: *(i)* the psychosomatic factors, such as nervousness, tension and various forms of stress and strain; and *(ii)* improper eating habits, such as over-eating, eating at irregular hours, going to bed immediately after the evening meal, not eating a balanced diet, excessive use of hot spices and fried things, eating adulterated or stale food stuffs, not chewing the food properly, unhygienic ways of eating, etc.

We have found that these disorder are easily relieved through the yoga system of treatment. In most of the cases, the trouble is controlled within two weeks and usually eliminated in about two months. Let me explain how people suffering from these troubles can treat themselves by following the yoga system of practice.

The yoga system of treatment requires: *(i)* attention to diet, and *(ii)* daily practice of a few *asanas*. There are a few important points to remember about proper diet before describing the diet-chart.

Your Diet

Eat a balanced diet which means to include salad, green vegetables and fresh fruits along with the other dishes of the day. Eat at least two hours before going to bed at night. Do not drink during the meals, but only half an hour after finishing your meals. Take ten to twelve glasses of water every day. Avoid fried, roasted and spicy food. Exclude red-pepper, pickles, hot spices and chutney from your daily menu. Do not take more than two cups of tea or coffee in a day. If possible stop taking tea and coffee for a while. Also, avoid drinking aerated drinks. Drinking water on arising in the morning should stop. Non-vegetarians can take fish or liver but should avoid any other meat for a while. People with any kind of abdominal disorder should eat according to the diet-chart given below:

Breakfast (7 to 9 a.m.)
(i) Choice of: any fruit juice or vegetable juice
    – half glass

(ii) Choice of: any fresh sweet fruit which is
     easily digestible such as, peaches, grapes,
     apples and pears.

(iii) Toast (wheat bread) – one or two slices or
      muffins with butter or choice of: Oatmeal or
      cornmeal with butter.

(iv) Egg (poached, medium boiled or
     scrambled).

(v) Tea, coffee, herbal – One cup tea or Ovaltine
    (if necessary)

Lunch (12 to 2 p.m.)
(i) Salad (a mixture of any three or more edible
    raw vegetables such as, tomato, cucumber,
    lettuce, radish, celery, carrot, beets, water-
    cress, onions etc.) taken with salad-dressing,
    vinegar oil dressing or cottage cheese.

(ii) Vegetable soup of any kind.

(iii) Wheat bread or corn bread or rice.

(iv) Stew of any kind of green and fresh veg-
     etables.

(v) Spinach or broccoli.

(vi) Dessert: Melon, Fresh berries or custard.

Afternoon Snack (3 to 5 p.m.)

(i) Fresh fruit in season.

(ii) Salted biscuits and cheese or choice of: Mixture of raw nuts (cashews, almonds, pecans, pistachios, walnuts).

(iii) Coffee, tea, herbal – one cup tea or Ovaltine (if necessary)

Dinner (7 to 9 p.m.)
(i) Mixed salad with salad-dressing or cole slaw.
(ii) Vegetable soup or broth.

(iii) Wheat bread.

(iv) Baked potato.

(v) Broiled fish, sea-food or liver.

(vi) Green vegetables (steamed or stewed)

(vii) Dessert: fruit cup, melon, or custard.

Yoga Practice
The important pranayama and asanas for correcting these disorders are: *Pranayama* with *Rechaka* and *Pooraka*, *Uttanpada asana*, *Pawanmukta asana*, *Bhujanga asana*, *Shalabha asana*, *Paschimottan asana*, and *Shava asana*.

The method of practising these asanas and the Pranayama are comprehensively described and illustrated in the following pages:

PRANAYAMA (with Rechaka and Pooraka)
Pranayama is a special form of exercise. There are various forms of *Pranayama*. Though each form is done differently, most of them have the following three steps in common:

  Rechaka (exhalation)
  Pooraka (inhalation)
  Kumbaka (retention)

In this particular *pranayama*, there are only *rechaka* and *puraka* but no *kumbaka* (retention of the breath). One significant aspect of this *pranayama* is that it is a diaphragmatic breathing. In this exercise the stomach is pulled in and out in a rhythmic way. It is very important to remember that the stomach is not pushed upward and downward.

Position of Readiness: Sit on the floor either in *Padmasana* (Lotus pose) as shown in Fig. 1, or in *Sukhasana* (Easy pose) as shown in Fig. 2. Hold the spine, neck and head absolutely erect. Look straight ahead. Stretch your arms and rest your wrists on the knees. Bring your thumb and index finger of each hand to meet together so that they form a circle and keep the other three fingers opened straight and joined together. Breathe normally.

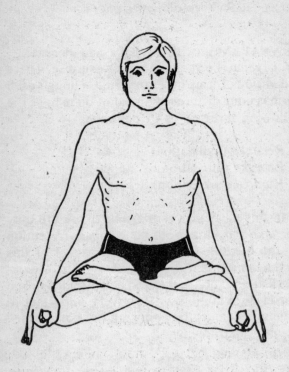

Fig. 1 *Padmasana.*

Steps of Actual practice: (i) Exhale slowly through both nostrils and simultaneously pull your stomach inwards, i.e. contract the abdominal muscles to expel air from your lungs. Keep exhaling till all the air is expelled from your lungs.

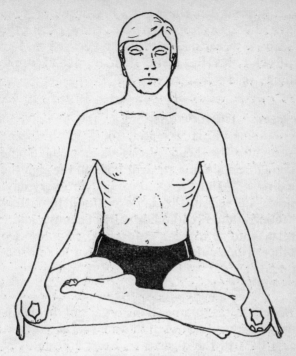

Fig. 2 *Sukhasana.*

(ii) Having exhaled, hold yourself in that position for a second and then slowly start inhaling through both nostrils. Inhale as deeply as you can by stretching out the abdominal muscles. The expansion of the stomach with inhalation should be gradual and rhythmical, not abrupt and fast.

(iii) After inhaling deeply, pause for a second and then start exhaling again. Continue this process ten to fifteen times (one exhalation and one inhalation each time).

Daily Practice: During the first week of practice, do this exercise ten times daily. During the second week and afterwards, increase it to fifteen times. But do not do it more than fifteen times in a single day.

Special Attention: As long as this *pranayama* continues, it is essential to keep the spine straight. The head, the neck and the spine should remain in a straight line, all through the exercise. After the exercise is over every day, hold yourself in the same position for a few seconds, and breathe normally. Then gradually relax into a more comfortable position. Do other *asanas* after waiting for five to ten seconds.

Benefits: It activates all the organs of the digestive system. Because of this internal activation, disorders of the digestive system are removed and corrected. Problems like constipation, dysentery, diarrhoea, gastric, indigestion and stomach ache are corrected.

This *pranayama* also affects various glands of the endocrine system. The adrenal, pancreas, ovaries in female and testicles in male are specifically activated and energized. Because of their internal activation, these glands begin to secrete respective hormones in a normal way.

It also corrects disorders of the circulatory and respiratory systems. It is an easy *pranayama* and can be practised by any person without any difficulty.

UTTANPADA ASANA

Position of Readiness: Lie with your back on the floor and look upwards at the ceiling. Keep both the arms straight alongside the body with palms touching the floor. Straighten both the legs and join your heels and toes. Breathe normally.

Steps of Actual Practice: (i) Inhale slowly but deeply through both nostrils and hold the breath.

(ii) Stretch out your toes as much as you can.

(iii) Slowly lift both legs up, about ten to twelve inches high from the floor and keep them there for six to eight seconds while holding the breath as shown in Fig. 3.

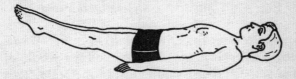

Fig. 3 *Uttanpada asana.*

(iv) Then start exhaling and lowering the legs towards the floor, both acts so synchronized that the legs reach the floor as you finish exhaling.

(v) Now rest for two normal breaths which should take about five to six seconds.

(vi) After resting, repeat the process.

Daily practice: Do it four times daily. Do not practice more than five times in a single day.

Note: Those people who have ever had any back injury or are otherwise weak, should not do this *asana* with both legs. They are advised to practise *Uttanpada asana* with one leg only, at a time (as shown in Fig. 4), till they get used to its impact. After practising with one leg at a time for about four weeks, they may start with both legs together.

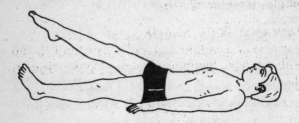

Fig. 4 *Uttanpada asana with one leg.*

The reason for this precaution is that *Uttanpada asana* brings great strain on the whole of the spine and also on the rest of the body. This strain is cut to half by doing the *asana* with one leg only. The process of doing it with one leg is the same as for doing it with both legs. The only difference is that instead of lifting both legs together at a time, you have to lift only one leg and leave the other on the floor. Do it alternately, with the other leg, completing three times with each leg. Do not practise for more than six times at a stretch.

Benefits of Uttanpada: This *asana* exercises all the abdominal muscles, both internally and externally. As a result, this *asana* corrects the disorders of the pancreas and relieves constipation, wind troubles, indigestion and intestinal disorders. It takes away the extra weight of the abdominal area.

This *asana* also has a great curative and corrective effect on aches in the back, waist, buttocks or hip-joints. It strengthens the spinal cord, energizes the inner cells and activates the whole nervous system.

PAWANMUKTA ASANA
Position of Readiness: Stand on the floor. Keep both hands hanging down. Look straight ahead.

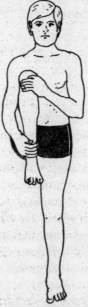

Fig. 5 *Pawanmukta asana.*

Steps of Actual Practice: (i) Lift right knee up towards the chest.

(ii) Put the right hand on the ankle and the other hand on the knee as shown in Fig. 5.

(iii) Pull the knee towards the chest without pulling on the ankle.

(iv) Stand firmly on the other leg, keeping quite straight.

(v) Stay in that position for six to eight seconds then release the knee and put the foot on the floor.

(vi) Rest for six seconds and repeat the same process with the other leg.

Daily Practice: Do it six to eight times daily (three to four times with each knee alternately).

Note: Those who experience difficulty in performing this *asana* in the standing position, may do it lying on the back. Method of practice remains the same as in the standing position.

Benefits: It activates the pancreas and other organs of the abdomen in a mild effective way. It is also a wind reliever. For people suffering from wind trouble, acidity and gas formation, it has an instant corrective effect. It loosens the hip joints and activates the whole of the abdominal muscles and intestines. As a result of its internal activation, it relieves constipation, and corrects any malfunctioning of the stomach. Because of this internal effect it helps to restore the functioning of the pancreas. It is an easy and harmless *asana.* Any person can do it.

BHUJANGASANA

Position of Readiness: Lie on stomach. Let the head rest on cheek. Bring the palms beneath the shoulders on both sides. Bring the tips of the finger to the edge of shoulders, elbows should be bent close to the body. Keep the heels together and the toes flat on the floor. Breathe normally.

Steps of Actual Practice: (i) Straighten the head and tilt it slightly backward.

(ii) Inhaling slowly, raise your head and chest upwards so that while your navel is on the floor, the portion above the navel is raised up. In this position both legs should be fully stretched and kept tightly together as shown in Fig. 6.

(iii) Then look up into the sky and hold your breath for six to eight seconds.

(iv) After six to eight seconds, start exhaling and lowering the head towards the floor and let the head rest on any cheek.

(v) Now let the body relax and rest for six seconds.

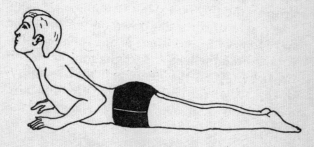

Fig. 6 *Bhujangasana.*

(vi) After a rest, repeat the process.

Daily Practice: Four times only.

Benefits: Bhujangasana inwardly activates the whole of the abdominal area. Because of this activation, the pancreas, liver and other organs of the digestive system are strengthened and normalized. It is regarded as one of the best *asanas* for alleviating constipation, indigestion, dysentry, wind troubles, stomach ache and other abdominal disorders. It brings flexibility to the spine and corrects spinal disorders and backache. It activates chest, shoulder, neck, face and head areas in an effective way and enhances facial beauty.

It has some specific benefits for women. Various menstrual problems are corrected by this *asana*.

SALABHASANA

Position of Readiness: Lie down on your stomach. Put any cheek on the floor. Stretch the hands on both sides of the body and keep them close to the thighs. Keep the thumb and index finger side of the palm down on the floor and make fists with both hands in the same position. Stretch both the legs and let the toes lie flat on the floor. Keep the heels and toes together. Make the whole body straight. Breathe normally. Now you are ready for making the *asana*.

Steps of Actual Practice: (i) Inhale slowly but

deeply through both nostrils and hold the breath.

(ii) Lift the head slightly, make it straight and then let the chin rest on the floor (use a folded towel underneath the chin).

(iii) Make the fists firm and tighten the arms and the hands.

(iv) Now tighten both the legs together and lift them up quickly as high as you can.

(v) Stay in that position for five to six seconds, or less, keeping the legs tensed (as shown in Fig. 7).

(vi) Then slowly exhale, simultaneously lowering the legs down towards the floor.

(vii) When the legs have touched the floor, turn the head to let it rest on the either cheek and let the whole body relax.

(viii) Rest for five seconds then repeat the *asana* in the same order as before.

Daily Practice: Repeat it only four times daily. (Do it after performing the *Bhujangasana* four times.)

Note: Those who might feel difficulty in lifting both legs together are advised to lift only one leg at a time (as shown in Fig. 8) for a few weeks. In this case, practise six rounds alternating each leg every time.

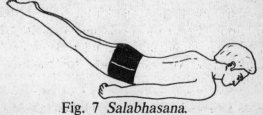

Fig. 7 *Salabhasana.*

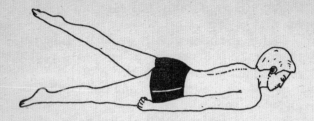

Fig. 8 *Salabhasana with one leg at a time.*

Benefits: It has a curative effect on various abdominal troubles. It activates the kidneys, the liver, pancreas, and the whole of the abdominal area. Because of internal activation, it removes constipation, wind troubles, indigestion, dysentery, diarrhoea, acidity and gastrointestinal disorders.

This *asana* has also various other good effects on the body as a whole. It brings flexibility to the spine and invigorates the eyes, the face, lungs, chest, neck, shoulders and the whole upper area of the body. Since it is a harmless *asana* it is recommended for everyone.

PASCHIMOTTANASANA
Position of Readiness: Sit on the floor and stretch both your legs in front. Keep the heels and toes together. Be seated firmly, keeping the spine, neck and head straight upward. At this stage, keep the hands down on the floor on both sides.

Steps of Actual Practice: (i) Stretch out both hands parallel with the stretched legs.

(*ii*) Touch the right toe with the right-hand fingers and the left toe with the left-hand fingers (as shown in Fig. 9). In case you cannot touch the toes, go only as far as possible while keeping both the legs stretched and palms down. Do not bend or lift the knees.

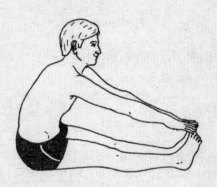

Fig. 9 *Readiness for Paschimottanasana.*

(*iii*) Bow your head downwards till it comes between the arms. Exhale all air out by the time the head is down.

(*iv*) Now stretch the toes and tense the legs, and while keeping the head between the arms, stretch both hands as far forward as possible. Without bending the legs, stay in that position for six to eight seconds (see Fig. 10)

(*v*) Now drop both palms on the legs and start inhaling and returning to the position of readiness. Let the palms drag back over the legs while returning.

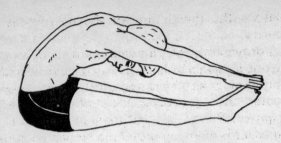

Fig. 10 *Paschimottanasana.*

(vi) Rest for five seconds and repeat the process.

Daily Practice: Do it four times daily. (Practise at least three times and at most five times a day.)

Note: Those who have back injury or spinal disorders with severe pain are advised to practise lightly and comfortably without forcing the body to bend excessively.

Benefits: This *asana* has an effect on the whole of the spinal cord, the complete nervous system and all the organs and glands of the abdominal area. As a result of these actions, disorders of these parts can be corrected. For diabetic people it has a beneficial effect because it activates the pancreas and the glands of the endocrine system. This internal action regularizes the functioning of the pancreas and it begins to secrete insulin in a normal way.

This *asana* also has several other good results. It corrects backache, alleviates spinal disorders, relieves stomach troubles, and normalizes the functioning of the nervous system.

For many people, it might not be possible to do this *asana* accurately. They are advised to do only as much as they can comfortably do. In due course, after practising for a while, they will improve. Remember that the method of doing an *asana* is more important than repeating it for a number of times. Since it is a very beneficial *asana*, it is recommended to everyone.

SAVASANA

Position of Readiness: Lie down on your back. Keep the whole body loose and in a straight position. Palms can be either on the floor or you can keep them upwardly. Do not use any pillow under your head. At this point keep breathing in a normal way. Keep the eyes closed and let the whole body relax completely. This is the position of readiness and the same position remains during the actual practice (see Fig. 11).

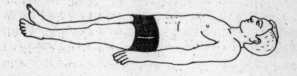

Fig. 11 *Savasana.*

Steps of Actual Practice: (i) Close your eyes and keep them closed for two seconds. Then open them for two seconds. Do this simple opening and closing of the eyes three or four times.

(ii) Open the eyes again and look upward, then downward, then straight ahead. Now look towards the left side, then towards the right side, then straight ahead again and then close the eyes. Repeat this eye exercise two to three times.

(iii) Now open your mouth widely without straining it. Turn the tongue so that the tip is folded back towards the throat area, then close the mouth. Keep the mouth closed and tongue folded for 10 seconds. Then open the mouth and bring the tongue back to its normal position, then close the mouth. Repeat the process two to three times.

(iv) Keeping your eyes closed, bring your mental attention towards your toes. See (mentally) that the toes are relaxed. Then move slowly upward and towards the head area mentally by checking the knees, thighs, waist, spinal cord, back, shoulders, neck, arms, palms, fingers and rest of the areas of the body to be sure that they are actually relaxed. Make a slight movement of the neck and head by turning right and left. Then let the head rest at a comfortable position. Now the entire body is physically relaxed.

(v) Then relax the mind with the following process:

Select a place of natural beauty which you have visited and liked, such as, a park, a garden, a lawn or a riverside and feel as if you are mentally present at that place. Attach your mind to that place. Feel as if you are lying in that place and breathing the air of the same environment. Now while keeping the mind involved with that environment, do some deep breathing. In this deep breathing, just exhale and inhale slowly but deeply. During the breathing, the stomach should go upward while inhaling and it should come downward while exhaling. One exhalation and one inhalation make one round. Do not rush in this deep breathing. Make about ten to twelve rounds. When the deep breathing is over, feel as if you are going to sleep. Now relax completely. Stay in that position for five to ten minutes. Then open your eyes and stretch your body and then be seated. You have completed the Savasana.

Daily Practice: Make *Savasana* at the end of all *asanas, pranayama* and other *Kriyas* for 10-15 minutes daily. In certain cases like hypertension and heart troubles, *Savasana* should be performed singly for longer periods without practising any *asana* or other *kriyas.*

Benefits: Savasana has a very beneficial effect upon people suffering from illness as well as those in good health. One immediate effect is that it relaxes all the muscles, nerves and the organs of the bodily system. When the muscles, nerves and organs are fully relaxed, they gain strength and their normal health is restored.

For the people suffering from insomnia, high and low blood pressure, gastric troubles, lung and heart troubles and mental sickness. *Savasana* is a remarkable *kriya* for providing immediate relief. Those who feel lack of energy, tiredness and fatigue will find this *asana* a giver of energy and strength. Because of these good effects, every practiser of Yoga is advised to practise it.

3.

Diabetes

This chapter deals with the treatment of those suffering from diabetes. We know that diabetes is a very old disease and millions all over the world suffer from it. Though there are variations in the symptoms and nature of this disease, its common feature is the excessive sugar in the blood and its passing out with the urine of the sufferer. This excessive accumulation of sugar in the blood is caused by the malfunctioning of the pancreas.

When the pancreas — a gland situated in the upper side of the abdomen — does not produce enough insulin, the body fails to utilize sugar and create energy from it. In the absence of proper utilization of sugar, the body chemistry gets disturbed and the individual begins to develop various physical ailments and disorders. Consequently, there is frequent urination, excessive thirst, tiredness, loss of weight, blurring of vision, general weakness and skin disorders in diabetic patients. Further, hypertension (high blood pressure) and kidney disorders also develop. The orthodox method of treating the diabetic patient is to inject insulin to compensate what could not be produced by the pancreas.

The main trouble with medicinal treatment is that the patient has to keep taking injections and other medicines indefinitely and still the disease is not eliminated.

Yoga Treatment

The yoga system of treatment consists of two aspects: *(i)* proper diet, and *(ii)* regular yoga practice.

The yogic treatment restores the normal functioning of the pancreas and other glands of the endocrinal system. When these glands begin to function properly, the body chemistry becomes normal, and health is restored to normal level.

Relevant Asanas

Since the main problem here is to restore the normal functioning of the pancreas and some other glands, the first consideration is to select such *asanas* which can help to revive the normal functioning of the endocrinal system. Secondly, we should choose such *asanas* which are easily practised by all. Accordingly, the *asanas* we may recommend are: *Surya Namaskar asana, Uttanpada asana, Bhujanga asana, Shalabha asana, Paschimottan asana, Ardha*

Vakra asana, Matsyendra asana, Supta Vajra asana, Dhanu asana and *Shava asana*. A regular practice of even six to seven of these *asanas* would assist in the treatment of diabetes.

Diet for Diabetics
It is important for the persons suffering from diabetes to avoid fried, fatty, spicy, starchy and sugar containing food. For a period of four months from the date of starting yoga practices, diabetic patients *should not take* rice, potatoes bananas, grapes, oranges, mangoes and such fruits in which the percentage of sugar is high. Diabetics should eat sprouted grams and cheese. They can take an apple a day. The non-vegetarians can add small quantities of fish, liver and eggs to their diet but should avoid meat or chicken for a few months.

Breakfast (7 to 9 a.m.)
(i) Vegetable juice — half a glass or tomato juice

(ii) Fresh apple — one or half.

(iii) Sprouted grams — 1/4 cup (about a (chickpeas)   handful)

(iv) Whole wheat — one or two slices bread or toast or Muffin without butter or choice of:

Oatmeal/cornmeal with milk.

(v) Egg (poached, medium-boiled or scrambled)

(vi) Tea/coffee/herbal tea/without sugar — one cup (if necessary)

Lunch and Dinner (12 to 2 p.m.: 8 p.m.)

(i) Salad (a mixture of cucumber, lettuce, radish, celery, watercress, tomato, onions) — taken with vinegar and oil dressing or salad dressing.

(ii) Soup or broth : Vegetable or bean soup or broth of any kind.

(iii) Wheat bread.

(iv) Broiled fish/sea-food/or liver.

(v) Steamed or stewed green vegetables of any kind.

(vi) Yogurt or cottage — (if desired) cheese

Afternoon Snacks (3 to 5 p.m.)

(i) Any fresh fruit

(ii) Salted biscuits or choice of:

Raw nuts (cashew, almond, pecan, walnuts): a handful of a mixture of these nuts taken from the hard shells and unroasted.

(iii) Tea, coffee, or herbal tea without sugar.

SURYANAMASKAR ASANA

Starting Position: Stand up keeping the legs about two feet apart. Let the hands hang loosely at the sides. Keep the head straight. Look straight ahead and breathe normally.

Steps of Actual Practice: (i) Inhale slowly and raise both hands upwards, in a sideways circular movement. Time it in such a way that by the time your hands come up, you also complete inhaling. When the hands are up, the palms should be turned forward and the arms should be parallel with each other.

(ii) Start exhaling and lowering the upper area of the body towards the ground. While thus bending forward, keep both hands parallel to one another and move them towards the ground, in a circular motion in front of you. By the time both hands reach near the floor, you should finish exhaling.

(iii) Now hold the breath and stay in that position for about six to eight seconds. While holding your breath, it is important that you keep the upper part of the body (above the waist) quite relaxed, and the lower part, i.e. the waist, rigid and hard. Bend your head down towards the ground. Your head should be between the two arms. Hands should be loosely hanging as far down as they can easily go. If you can bend easily, put the palms on the floor or just touch the floor. It is important that you are not straining yourself or forcing your body excessively. Do only as much as you can comfortably(see Fig. 12).

(iv) Bring both hands to the legs and inhale and come up in the standing position. While coming up let the palms pass over and touch the legs upwardly. Inhale slowly in such a way that by the time you have returned to the standing position you have finished inhaling. Now you have completed one round of *Suryanamaskar asana.*

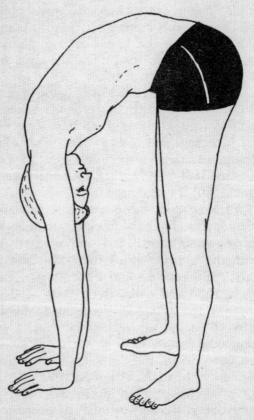

Fig. 12 *Suryanamaskar asana*

(v) Rest five to six seconds and then repeat the same process. Stay in the position of readiness while resting.

Daily Practice: Practice four times daily. Do not do it more than four times in a single day.

Benefits: This *asana* has several good benefits. It activates almost all the glands of the endocrinal system gently. Because of this internal activation, the pancreas, adrenal, thyroid, pituitary and some other glands begin to secrete their respective hormone in a normal way. Since the main trouble with persons of diabetic disorder results from the malfunctioning of the pancreas, this *asana* corrects its defects by activating it.

It has a good effect on the stomach, spine, lungs and chest. Various disorders of these areas are corrected by this *asana*. As there is reverse circulation of blood during this *asana*, it invigorates the facial tissues, the central nerve system and all the organs of the upper part of the body. It is easy to do and therefore recommended to all practisers of Yoga.

After practising *Suryanamaskar asana*, the following *asana* should be gradually added to daily practice.

Uttanpada asana (See Figs. 3 and 4)
Bhujangasana (See Fig. 6)
Salabhasana (See Figs. 7 and 8)
Paschimottasana (See Figs. 9 and 10)

All the above-mentioned four *asana* are fully described in chapter 2 (under the heading 'Abdominal Disorders'). The diabetic patients are advised to practise these *asanas* according to the method described there.

ARDHAVAKRA ASANA

Position of Readiness: Sit down on the floor. Stretch both legs in front. Make the legs parallel to one another. Put both palms on the floor. Breathe normally. Keep the back straight while sitting.

Steps of Actual Practice: (i) Let one leg remain stretched on the floor. Bend the other leg and pull it slightly backward.

(ii) Place the heel of the bent leg at the central point between the knee and the ankle of the stretched leg on the outer side of the leg. Keep the heel quite close to the stretched leg. Now the knee of your folded leg should be pointing upward.

(iii) Lift the hand which is on the side of the stretched leg; bring it up and parallel to the stretched leg. Grab the stretched leg near the heel of the bent leg. Now you have made a lock with the arm and the knee. If you cannot grab the stretched leg, just touch it or keep the fingers near the central point.

(iv) Lift the hand on the other side and put the palm on the waist, keeping the thumb and the index finger side upward. At this stage see that your head, neck and back are straight.

(v) Start exhaling slowly and at the same time begin twisting and turning the waist, chest, neck and the head area in the direction of the bent elbow. Twist and turn as far as you can go comfortably. In this turn, your folded elbow travels 90 degrees but the head and the upper area of the body travel 180 degrees. For example, if you were sitting facing east and you have to turn to the right side then your face will turn first to south and then to the west side while your stretched leg will remain facing east.

(vi) After making the maximum turn, hold the breath and stay in that position for six to eight seconds. At this stage, your spine should be straight and you should be projecting the vision at a maximum distance (as shown in Fig. 13).

(vii) Then start inhaling slowly and return to the position of readiness.

(viii) Now break the lock, stretch out the legs, relax the body, put the palms on the floor and rest for six seconds.

(ix) After the rest repeat the *asana* with the other leg, following the same method.

Daily Practice: Make four to six rounds alternately. Never do it more than six times (three times with each side).

Benefits: The main beneficial effect of this *asana* is on the waist and abdominal areas. It activates all the organs and glands of these parts of the body. This *asana* has a very good effect on the pancreas, adrenal, ovary in female and the testicle in male.

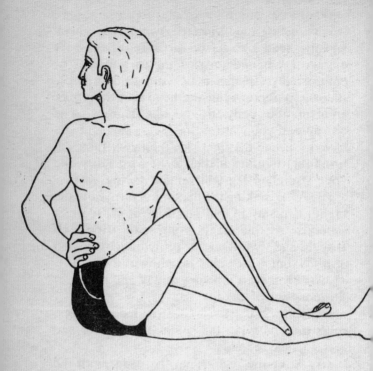

Fig. 13 *Ardhavakra asana.*

It has several other beneficial effects. It corrects constipation, stomach troubles, piles, backache, stiffness in the neck and spinal disorders. It is easy to do and therefore recommended to every practiser of yoga.

MATSYENDRASANA

Matsyendrasana is a little difficult. It may not be possible for everyone to do it perfectly in the beginning. But since it is an important *asana*, the practisers are advised to do it only as much as they can quite comfortably. Those people who can practise *Matsyendrasana* perfectly well should not practise *Ardhavakra asana* as both have a similar effect. Since *Ardhavakra asana* is easier to do, the practisers should begin with it first.

Position of Readiness: Be seated on the floor. Stretch both legs in front. Keep the legs parallel. Put the palms on the floor on both sides of the body. Make the body straight. Look in front and breathe normally.

Steps of Actual Practice: *(i)* Bend the right leg at the knee by pulling it backward. Now the right thigh is standing upward and the right side buttock has been raised up. At this stage, keep this right leg where it is.

(ii) Bend the left leg at the knee without lifting it up. The thigh and knee of the left leg should remain on the floor and the foot should be brought below the right buttock. The left foot may be gently pulled in order to bring it underneath the buttock.

(iii) Now lift the right foot slightly up and bring it on the outer side of the left knee. Keep the right foot bent. Now your right knee is standing up and the left knee is down on the floor

(iv) Stretch out the left arm and bring it on the

outer side of the right knee. Lock your arm against the standing knee firmly. Grab the right foot with the left hand in order to provide stability

(v) Keep the whole of the right arm and hand at the back relaxed. Try to touch the front part of the waist with the fingers of the hand at the back. You are now ready for making the turn. At this stage see that your backbone, neck and head are in a straight upward position.

(vi) Now start exhaling slowly and turning the head, chest and waist towards the right side. Twist the body as much as you can. Be sure that all air has been thrown out by the time you have made the full twist. Look at the farthest distance possible. Keep the back straight upward. You should be as in Fig. 14.

(vii) Stay in the position for six to eight seconds. The holding time may be for only four to six seconds in the beginning stage of practice.

(viii) Then start inhaling slowly and gradually return to the position from where you had started the twist. You have completed one round of *Matsyendrasana*.

(ix) Now unlock the arm and the knee and be seated in the position of readiness and rest for six to eight seconds. During the rest just inhale and exhale deeply twice.

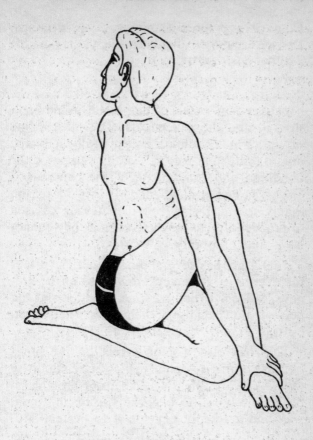

Fig. 14 *Matsyendrasana*

(x) After the rest be prepared for turning to the
left side in another round. Now your left knee
will be standing up and your right arm will be
locked. Keep doing it alternately.

Daily Practice: Make four to six rounds daily

Do not ever practise it for more than six rounds. Do it alternately and only as much as is possible without undue strain.

Benefits: This *asana* has a great effect on the pancreas and other glands, such as adrenal, thyroid and the sex glands. The muscle and organs of the abdominal area are fully activated due to this *asana*. Because of this activation the condition and functioning of the pancreas is energized and strengthened. This is the reason that people suffering from diabetes are advised to practise this *asana* daily even if they cannot do it quite properly.

This *asana* has several other beneficial effect for everyone. It corrects disorders of the kidneys, spleen, liver, intestine, bladder and the pelvis region because of their internal activation by this *asana*

This has also a good effect on the lungs because of improvement in blood circulation by this *asana*. People suffering from breathlessness are advised to begin this *asana* in a mild way and gradually develop it to perfection.

This *asana* has some specific benefits in cases of spinal disorders. It removes rigidity of the spine and restores flexibility in it. Since it twists the whole of the spinal cord from the cervix to the coccyx in an effective and mild way disorders of the whole spine are corrected.

Since it is a very beneficial *asana* for diabetic people as well as for others, everyone is advised to do it.

SUPTAVAJRASANA

Position of Readiness: Sit on the floor with your legs folded under you. (See Fig 15.) Put the palms on the floor on both sides of the body and straighten your spine. Now look in front and breathe normally.

Note: This *asana* is a little difficult. Those whose body condition is not very flexible are advised to practise this *asana* in a gradual way without trying to do the complete *asana* all at once. By doing it in stages, it can be done without any strain.

Steps of Actual Practice: (i) Kneel on the floor, keeping the body weight on both the knees. Put the palms on the floor on each side of the folded knees to support part of the body weight. Keep the knees about four inches apart from one another. Let the ankles and toes of both the legs fall on the floor in such a way that the toes are brought close together but the heels are spread out. This will make a "V" curve with the toes, soles and the heels.

(ii) Now gradually and cautiously start lowering the hips and let them rest on the curve of the soles. Control the body weight by keeping both hands on the floor while lowering the hips. If you do not feel strained, put the whole body weight on the curve of the feet as shown in Fig. 15. In case of difficulty in sitting in this position, further stages should not be tried till the body is prepared for it. Those who can sit comfortably on the toes and soles should proceed to the third stage.

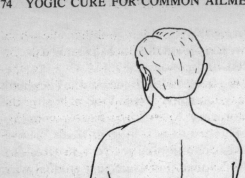

Fig. 15 *Back view of sitting position for making Suptavajrasana*

(iii) Lift the right hand and place it on the floor behind the hip. Then move the left hand also behind the hip and bend a little backward.

(iv) Now put the right elbow on the floor while bending backward. Then put the left elbow on the floor. By moving the elbows towards the hips gradually let the head touch the floor. When the head has come on the ground,

gradually put the shoulders and then the whole back of your body on the floor. Do not rush. Go slow in this process.

(v) Now stretch both the arms and hands on both sides of the body. Keep the palms on the floor and in close to the body, as shown in Fig. 16.

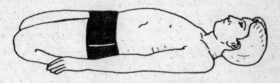

Fig. 16 *Suptavajrasana*

(vi) Then do a few deep breathings by just inhaling and exhaling the air through both nostrils. Stay in that position for six to eight seconds or less. You are in *Suptavajrasana.*

(vii) Now you have to return with the following method: Grab the ankles with the hands and put the elbows on the floor. Now pull the ankles and by putting the weight of the body on the elbows lift the head and back and return to the sitting position.

(viii) Then outstretch the bent leg and be seated in the position of readiness for a rest.

(ix) Rest for six to eight seconds and then repeat the *asana* with the same process.

Daily Practice: Do it three to four times. Never do it more than five times.

Benefits: This *asana* has some specific benefits for people suffering from diabetes. Since this *asana* activates all the cells of pancreas and increases its blood supply, it begins to function in a normal way. This *asana* has several other benefits. It corrects disorders of stomach, intestine, liver, kidneys, spleen and all the organs of the abdominal area by activating and energizing them.

It has medicinal value for people suffering from indigestion, wind trouble, constipation and piles. The disorders of the spine and joints are effectively corrected by this *asana*. It also has a good effect on the sex glands. It enhances sexual potentiality.

DHANURASANA

Position of Readiness: Lie down on your stomach. Keep your arms stretched on both sides. Place your head resting on any cheek on the floor. Bring the legs and heels together. Breathe normally. Bend both the legs at the knees and bring the heels close to your hips. Then grab the right ankle with the right hand and the left ankle with the left hand. In case you find it difficult to reach the ankles, you may hold the toes. Now holding either the ankles or the toes firmly, bring the knees and the ankles close together. Keep the cheek on the floor. You are now in position for performing *Dhanurasana*.

Steps of Actual Practice: (i) Inhale slowly but deeply and hold the breath.

(ii) When the inhaling is over, lift the head up and straighten it.

(iii) Give a backward pull with both the legs.

Do not rush in giving the backward pull. Do it slowly but constantly and smoothly. Let the legs fly out backwards as far as they can go. This will raise your chest, neck and head upward.

(iv) Look towards the sky, keep the knees close to one another and on the floor. Do not lift the knees up from the floor. Keep the ankles together, if possible. Remain in this position for six to eight seconds while holding the breath. You should be as in Fig. 17.

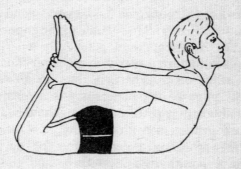

Fig. 17 *Dhanurasana*

(v) Start exhaling and simultaneously lowering the head and chest towards the floor.

(vi) Let your head rest on the floor, on either cheek, and also release the ankles and let them fall back slowly on the floor. Bring the hands also on the floor and relax. You have completed one round of *Dhanurasana*.

(vii) After resting for six to eight seconds, repeat the *asana* with the same process as done during the first round.

Daily Practice: Do it three to four times only. Those who might find it difficult to do the complete *asana* by holding both the ankles are advised to practise for a few days with only one ankle at a time.

In this case, the whole process of inhaling, raising up, holding and returning remains the same as done with both ankles. The only difference is that one leg remains stretched on the floor while the other is bent, held and pulled. It is very easy to do with one ankle at a time.

Benefits: Dhanurasana has several good benefits. It activates all the glands of the endocrinal system. The pancreas gets fully energized because of internal as well as external impact of this *asana* on it. There is thus an all round conditioning of the pancreas. As a result, its normal health is restored and it should begin to release insulin in a proper way.

The *asana* has a good effect on adrenal, thyroid, parathyroids, pituitary and the sex glands. Since the cells of all these glands are activated, the secretion of their respective hormones become normal.

It has corrective effects on the disorders of the joints, spinal cord, lungs, chest and abdomen. It removes various types of stomach troubles, develops digestive power and takes off extra weight and fat.

The *asana* has some specific benefits for women. It corrects menstrual disorders and other troubles related to the reproductive organs.

4.

Asthma

The main trouble with asthma is breathlessness. The breathless condition of the patient is caused by the disorder and bronchial spasm in the respiratory system.

The most common symptom of this disease is that the patient feels difficulty in breathing. There is a strain in exhaling the air. The asthmatic has to try hard in order to draw a single breath. In severe cases, the life of the patient becomes miserable and it makes him almost invalid. In medical terms the complicated condition of asthma is called emphysema.

Asthma is mainly a disorder of the bronchioles. There is constriction of the bronchioles which disturbs the normal ratio of inspiration and expiration. Because of congestion of the blood vessels of the bronchial lining the expiration begins to get prolonged and difficult.

It is a widely prevalent disease of our time,

affecting the young, old and even the children. In our country, millions suffer from this tortuous disease. The most disheartening aspect of asthma is that it does not get completely cured through medicine.

In treating the patients of asthma at the Indian institute of yoga, Patna, we have found a very satisfactory result. The patients who followed our instructions well and practised yoga regularly enjoyed improved health. We noticed that the health of both male and female patients became normal within a few months of this yoga practice and that there was no recurrence of it once the treatment had succeeded.

The system of treatment of this disease necessitates three things: *(i)* regular practice of *pranayama* and selected *asanas, (ii)* eating a proper diet, *(iii)* observance to certain principles and advices. Let me explain these aspects.

PRANAYAMA AND ASANAS

The selection of *pranayama* and *asanas* is made according to the need of the body in this disease. As already mentioned above, the disease is primarily of the lungs and the respiratory system. Therefore, the *pranayama* and *asanas* have to be so selected as their practice would restore the normal health of the lungs and the whole of the respiratory system. Keeping this aim in view the following *pranayama* and *asanas* are recommended:

UJJAYI PRANAYAMA

Ekpadauttan asana; Tara asana; Yoga Mudra; Ushtra asana; Simhasana; Sarvangasana; Matsyasana; Padmasana and *Shavasana.*

The process of practising them will be presented one by one in the following pages.

Proper Diet for Asthmatics

The asthmatics should eat a balanced diet which means including salad, fresh fruits, green vegetables, germinated gram and leafy vegetables in their daily meals. They should eat four times a day, that is, breakfast, lunch, some sort of afternoon refreshment and dinner.

Breakfast should consist of some fruit juice, fresh fruits, a handful of germinated gram, wheat bread and green vegetables.

The lunch and dinner should begin with salad (slices of cucumber, lettuce, tomato, carrot, beets, and any vegetable which can be eaten raw). Salad should be eaten, about a cupful mixed with salt, pepper and lemon juice or with salad dressing. This should be followed by soup (if possible), wheat bread, pulse and some fresh green vegetables. The non-vegetarians can eat fish and liver if they like, but any other sort of meat should be avoided for a period of three months.

In the afternoon, some light refreshment should be taken, such as fresh fruits, cheese, cake, or salted biscuits.

Points to Remember

It is most important that the asthmatics remember the following principles and advice in their diet and daily life. They must eat dinner at least two hours before going to bed at night. They should never eat to their full capacity at any time. They should eat slowly and chew the food properly, should drink water half an hour after finishing their meals, should take ten to twelve glasses of water in a day, and should avoid hot spices, red pepper and pickles. Their intake of tea or coffee should not be more than two cups in a day. They should not drink water upon arising and before going to toilet.

Asthmatics should avoid diet and such ways of living which they have found to be allergic. They are advised to cut down on or give up cigarettes, and the use of tobacco in any form. In case it is difficult to give up smoking, they should not smoke on an empty stomach. They should try to get six to eight hours sleep a night and should try to be relaxed rather than tensed. The conditions which cause nervousness and tension should be corrected and eliminated. The asthmatics are strongly advised to take a daily bath with soap and either cold or hot water, and to rub the whole body with a rough towel. They should avoid daily massaging the body with any oil. They should maintain neatness and cleanliness as much as possible. With these guidelines, they should practise the following *pranayamas* and *asanas*:

UJJAYI PRANAYAMA (IN LYING POSITION)

Pranayama is mainly a *kriya* (exercise) with air.

As we know air possesses several unique qualities. It contains (Prana shakti)life force. It also has an absorbing, activating and massaging capacity. Because of these qualities, the air is regarded as great purifier as well as a giver of life to the inner organs of the body. The body makes full use of these qualities of the air during Pranayama.

Ujjayee Pranayama can be practised in two ways: (i) in the standing position, and (ii)in the lying position. The full effect can be felt in the first position and a little less in the second position. But the first is a little strenuous and the second is the easiest. Therefore, the practisers are advised to practise Ujjayee in the lying position first for a period of one month and then may switch over to the standing position (as described next), if preferred.

Position of Readiness: Lie down on your back on the floor. Make the body straight. Put the palms on the floor and close to the body. Bring the heels together and keep the legs relaxed. Look straight upward. Breathe normally.

Steps of Actual Practice: There are altogether four steps in Ujjayi: (i)Exhaling the air through the mouth;

(ii) Inhaling the air through both nostrils;

(iii) Retaining the air; and

(iv) Exhaling the air again through the mouth. These steps have to be performed in a sequence as described below:

(i) Exhale all the air of the body through the

mouth quickly but steadily. The speed of air during exhalation is the same as it is when you whistle. The air is blown out through and between the lips without any twist on the facial tissues (see Fig. 18).

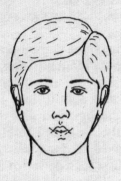

Fig. 18 *Showing Exhalation in Ujjayi Pranayama.*

During this stage, the body should remain relaxed. There should be contraction of the abdominal area while exhaling the air. When all the air has been exhaled, the second stage begins straight away.

(ii) Inhale air slowly with both nostrils. Do not rush. Let the air be filled in the body by as much as can be inhaled comfortably. Do not try to inhale excessively. Keep the body relaxed at this stage. The inhalation will make the abdominal area expanded.

(iii) When the inhalation is completed, retain the air inside and do the following steps: Bring the toes of both legs together and stretch them

forward. Tense the legs. Pull the stomach gradually inwards. Keep the hands stretched. There should be a mild tightening of the muscles of the whole body. Stay in this position (as shown in Fig. 19) for a period of three to four seconds only during the first week. Gradually increase the retaining time to six or eight seconds during the second or third week. The principle is to retain this position only for as long as you can quite comfortably.

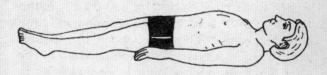

Fig. 19 *Retention in Ujjayi in lying position.*

(iv) After retaining for the desired seconds, exhale the air through the mouth in the same way as you did it during the first step. The air should be released steadily and continuously but in a controlled way. Do not rush. While exhaling, start relaxing the body muscles from the top downward; that is, first relax the chest, then the stomach, then the thighs, legs and the hands. Relax the whole body as you fully exhale. You have made one round of *Ujjayi Pranayama.* Now rest for five to six seconds.

During the rest just inhale and exhale through the nostrils. When the resting is over, repeat the same process as done during the first round.

Daily Practice: On the first day of your practice, perform it only three times. Increase to four times on the second day and then to five times on the third day. Do not do it more than five times at a stretch. That is the maximum at one time. Those who wish to practise it twice a day should wait for eight hours between the first and the second practice. Morning and evening times are the most suitable for practising twice a day.

Caution: *Pranayama* must be performed on an empty stomach. The best time to do it is in the morning, after washing. The second good time is in the evening. Those who would like to do it in the evening, must wait for three to four hours after lunch. It must be done where fresh air is available and when the body temperature is normal.

Benefits: Though a full description of its benefits is presented in the following pages, let me mention here that the practice of *Ujjayi Pranayama* in the lying position has all the benefits it has when done in the standing position. It is important to mention that it is safe and easy to do in the lying position for any person of any age and of any bodily condition. People with high blood pressure, low blood pressure, people in the habit of taking drugs, and people with heart trouble are specially advised to practise it in this position till they feel quite normal.

UJJAYI PRANAYAMA (IN STANDING POSITION)

The method of practising *Ujjayi Pranayama* in the lying position has been described earlier. Now the method of practising it whilst in the standing position is described. But first:- a word of warning.

Caution: *Ujjayi Pranayama* in the standing position must be practised according to the requirements and methods described herein. Any laxity in following the instructions can cause injury and harm to the practiser. Unless *Ujjayi Pranayama* in the standing position is practised properly, the practiser might fall over and injure himself. Therefore, it is advisable to obey the following guidelines while practising *Ujjayi Pranayama* in the standing position.

(i) Practise *Ujjayi Pranayama* first in the lying position for about a month, then try in the standing position. There is no danger of injury or harm in the lying position.

(ii) *Ujjayi Pranayama* in the standing position must be practised in fresh air, when the body is not tired, when the body temperature is normal, and when the practiser is not in a hurry.

(iii) Every step must be done gradually and rhythmically.

Position of Readiness: Standing up, join your heels and spread your toes at an angle of forty-five degrees to each other. Let the hands hang loosely at the sides. Look straight ahead. Stand firm but without tightening the body. Be cheerful.

Steps of Actual Practice. There are four steps in the standing position of *Ujjayi Pranayama. (i)* Exhaling air through mouth; *(ii)* Inhaling air through both nostrils, *(iii)* Retaining the air, and *(iv)* Exhaling the air again through the mouth. These four steps have to be done in the sequence described below:

(i) Exhale all air out through the mouth quickly but steadily. The air is blown out through the lips (see Fig. 18). The speed of exhaled air during this step is the same as it is when you whistle. During this stage keep the whole body relaxed. When you start exhaling, gradually pull the stomach muscles inside (contract the stomach). When all the air has been blown out, begin the second stage straight away.

(ii) Inhale slowly and continuously through both nostrils. Do not rush to finish inhaling quickly. Inhale without straining or twisting the facial muscles. Inhale only as much air as you can take quite comfortably. During inhalation, the body should remain relaxed. As the air fills the insides, the abdominal muscles should expand. In other words let the abdominal area expand in the same way as a balloon does when it is filled with air.

(iii) When the inhaling is over, retain (hold) the air inside. For retaining, it is important that you start tensing the whole body gradually from the legs upwardly to the chest. *Do not rush to retain all at once.* Run through the following process for the proper conditioning of your body during retention.

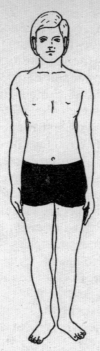

Fig. 20 *Retention in Ujjayi in standing position.*

First tighten the muscles of the legs and then tighten the muscles of the thighs. Now gradually pull the stomach in only as much as you can comfortably. Raise the chest slightly upwards. Bring the palms on the sides of the thighs and tense the hands and arms. Look straight ahead. Do not raise up the shoulders. Keep the whole body fairly tense. Do not tighten excessively. Retain the air inside for as long as you feel quite comfortable. Do not strain yourself too hard to hold the air, (see Fig. 20). At the beginning stage of practice hold your breath for two to three seconds only and gradually increase the holding time to six or eight seconds. Holding the breath for a very long time is not needed in *Ujjayi Pranayama*.

(iv) After holding the air for the specified time, exhale through the mouth steadily but quickly. Along with exhaling, gradually start relaxing the body from the chest downwards to the legs. First loosen the chest, then the abdominal muscles, then the thighs, legs and hands. By the time you have completely exhaled, the body should also become loose. While exhaling do not bend the head or chest either backward or forward. Keep standing in a straight position. With this, one round of *Ujjayi* is completed. Now rest for six to eight seconds. During the rest, just inhale and exhale twice through the nostrils while keeping the mouth closed. When the resting time is over, repeat the same process for further rounds.

Daily Practice: Begin with only three on the first day. Make four rounds on the second day and go to five rounds on the third day. Do not ever practise more than five rounds in a single session.

Benefits: The most remarkable benefit of *Ujjayi* is that it achieves internal purification, activation and energizing together with external control and conditioning all at the same time. For the asthmatics, *Ujjayi* is the most effective for correcting and strengthening the condition of the lungs and the bronchiole linings. In order

to convey its benefits properly let me explain
what Ujjayi does to the internal organs of the
body.

We know that air has an absorbing capacity.
It can absorb certain things such as moisture,
fragrance and odour. Air has also force and
power to carry things, such as, dust particles
and even heavier things. We also know that if
we put air in a balloon and give external pressure, the air would move and would try to
penetrate even the minutest available space.
With this understanding about the nature of air
it can easily be comprehended that when the air
is kept in the body for a longer time, it absorbs
the impurities of the system and when it is
expelled with a force it carries those inner
impurities out. Further, when external pressure
is given it maximizes the inner penetration of
the air and enables it to rub, activate and give
inner massage to the body cells and organs. This
inner massage is a unique benefit of Ujjayi and
is hence recommended highly for any adult
practiser of Yoga.

EKPADA UTTAN ASANA

In the preceding pages the methods of practising Ujjayi Pranayama have been fully
explained. The asthmatics have been advised to
practise five rounds of it daily in either the lying
or standing position. After doing Ujjayi the
asthmatics should practise the selected asanas
as presented in this chapter. The first asana of
this series is Ekpada uttan asana. Its method of

practice is explained below:

Position of Readiness: Lie down on your back on the floor. Make the body straight, bring the heels together. Keep the palms near to the body on the floor. Let the body remain relaxed. Look straight upwardly. Breathe normally.

Steps of Actual Practice: (i) Sretch out the toes of any one leg and make it hard and tight all along. Keep the other leg loose.

(ii) When the leg has been tightened, start inhaling and slowly raising it upwards. It should take about eight seconds to bring it upwardly in a perpendicular position. While lifting the leg upward do not twist or turn the other parts of the body. Let the whole body remain on the floor. Lift the leg only as high as it can go comfortably. Do not give excessive strain in pushing the leg upward.

(iii) When the leg has been brought to a maximum height, hold the breath and keep the leg in this position for six seconds only. During this stage of retention see that your body is straight; the lifted leg is quite tight, palms are down on the floor; and you are looking upwards as shown in Fig. 21.

(iv) After holding the breath for six seconds, start exhaling and lowering the leg towards the floor. It should take about eight seconds to complete exhalation. The leg should remain hard and tight while it is brought down. When the leg comes to the floor, one round of *Ekpada uttan asana* is completed.

(v) Now rest for six to eight seconds. After

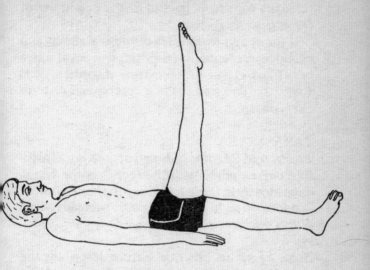

Fig. 21 *Ekpada uttan asana*

the resting time is over, start with the other leg by following the same process.

Daily Practice: Begin with four rounds. Do each leg alternately. Gradually increase to six rounds.

Benefits: For the asthmatics it has a curative effect. During retention the air penetrates the bronchioles and gently activates their linings.

This *asana* has several other benefits. It brings flexibilty to the hip joints and corrects disorders of the stomach and intestines. It removes wind troubles and gastric conditions of the digestive system.

It tones up the muscles of the sex-glands and enhances potentiality. For the women it has a beneficial effect on menstrual disorders. It is easy to do and hence recommended to everyone.

TARA ASANA
Position of Readiness: Stand up making a forty-five degree angle with the feet. Let the hands hang loosely at the sides. Keep the body straight and look straight ahead. Breathe normally. This is the position of readiness.

Steps of Actual Practice: Before describing the steps it needs to be pointed out that it is a *kriya* of the hands and the arms. In this *kriya* the hands are folded six times according to the following process:

(i) Tense the muscles of the hands and gradually raise them in front while inhaling. By the time the hands have been brought in front on the level of the shoulders, inhaling should be completed. Now hold the breath. Keep the palms facing upwards. Keep the hands straight, parallel and firm. This is the first fold as shown in Fig. 22.

(ii) After pausing for a second on the first fold, turn the palms downward and move the arms from the front to stretch out at the sides. During this second fold, let the hands come on the level of the shoulders in such a way that they

are in one line. Keep looking straight in front
while holding the breath(see Fig. 23).

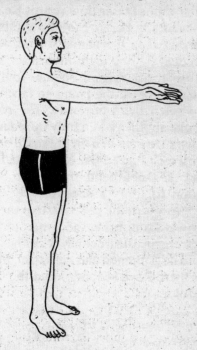

Fig. 22 *Hands in front for Tara asana.*

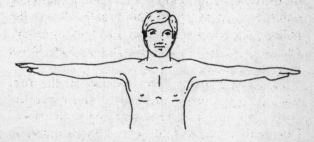

Fig. 23 *Hands at the sides in Tara asana.*

(iii) After pausing for a second on the second fold, bring the hands again in front while keeping the palms facing downward. Keep the hands tightened and parallel to one another. The distance between the hands should be six inches for teenagers and eight inches for adults. Give a pause for a second on this fold.

(iv) Then turn the palms to face one another and stretch them upwards. The palms should face one another when fully raised upwards and the distance between them should be six to eight inches(see Fig. 24). Keep looking straight ahead. Do not bend the body. Stay in that position for only a second.

(v) Now turn the palms so that they are facing downward and bring the hands to the sides as you were in the second fold(Fig. 23). Hands should be tightened and kept straight in one line. Stay there for a second. Hold the breath up to this fold.

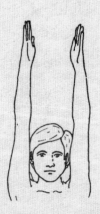

Fig. 24 *Hands up in Tara asana*

(vi) Then start exhaling and slowly lowering the hands. When the hands have returned to the sides, you should have exhaled completely.

Now relax the body and rest. Let the hands hang loosely. You have completed one round of *Tara asana*. After resting for two deep breaths make more rounds by following the same process.

Daily Practice: Do it only three times a day during the first week. During the second week and after, increase to four times daily. Five times should be the maximum in a day.

Benefits: Tara asana has a good strengthening effect upon the lungs and chest. Though the outward action in this *kriya* is of the hands, it internally activates the lungs, chest muscles and the respiratory system. For the asthmatics, therefore, it provides a corrective as well as a strengthening effect on their bronchioles and their lungs.

For those of sound health *Tara asana* has several good benefits. It increases the measurement of the chest. It builds up the muscles of the chest and has a curative effect for any disorder of that area.

Those who wish to add a few inches to their height might also find it very rewarding. People suffering from pain in their shoulder-joint can correct their disorders through *Tara asana*. It is easy to do. People of any age-group can do it.

YOGA MUDRA

Position of Readiness: The perfect way of practising *Yoga Mudra* is in the Lotus pose first. But
it is not easy for everyone to practise the Lotus
pose. Those who cannot do it properly should
sit on the floor with their legs crossed. After
being seated either in the Lotus or in *Sukhasana*
as shown in Fig. 1 and Fig. 2, do the following
steps, bring both the hands to the back. Hold the
wrist of one hand with the other hand. Make a
fist with the hand which is being held. At this
stage keep the hands loose and let them rest at
the back. Make the spine straight. Look in front
while keeping the neck and head straight
upwardly. This is the position of readiness.

Steps of Actual Practice: (i) Exhale gradually
and at the same time, start lowering the head
towards the earth. You have to synchronize
exhaling with the bending of the upper area of
the body towards the earth. Let the head come
down only as far as it can easily be lowered. Do
not put excessive strain on the spine while
lowering the head. If possible, touch the ground
with the forehead. By the time the head has
touched the ground all air should have been
completely exhaled.

(ii) After bending as far as possible retain the
breath. Now tense the hands and gradually raise
them (still with one hand holding the wrist of the
other) upwards as high as possible without
giving excessive strain. Remain in this position
for six to eight seconds as shown in Fig. 25.

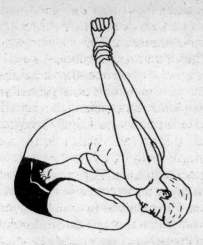

Fig. 25 *Yoga Mudra.*

(iii) Start inhaling while lowering the hands and gradually return to the position of readiness. Relax the hands and the body. Rest for six to eight seconds. After resting, repeat the process a few more times.

Daily Practice: Make only two rounds daily during the first week and increase it to four rounds during the second week. Its four rounds are the *maximum*.

Benefits: It activates and exercises the lungs in a very effective way. Because of the reverse position of the upper area of the body, the blood from the lower region begins to flow upwards and thereby massages the veins of the lower bronchioles of the lungs. This helps restore the normal health of the lungs and their functioning. For these reasons *Yoga Mudra* has a beneficial effect for asthmatics.

For the general purposes, *Yoga Mudra* provides several good benefits. It helps correct orders of the spine; removes gastric troubles and constipation; strengthens the digestive system; and enhances sexual potentiality.

USHTRA ASANA
Position of Readiness: You need to have something soft underneath the knees for performing this *asana*. Put a blanket or a towel on the floor. First be seated on the soft floor. Bend the legs and keep the knees about six inches apart. Then kneel down and let the ankles and toes of both legs lie flat on the floor. Keep the heels about six inches apart. Now the back of the knees, the calves and the heels would be in an upward position. This is the position of readiness for *Ushtra asana.*

Steps of Actual Practice: (i) Kneel and catch hold of the back of the ankles of the right leg with the right hand. Hold it firmly. If you cannot reach above the heel, you may just catch the heels.

(ii) Now catch hold of the left heel or the back of the left ankle with the left hand. Make the grip firm.

(iii) Holding the heels or the back of the ankles, straighten the thighs and waist. Bend the head and neck backwards as far as you can. Push the waist slightly forward. Breathe normally and stay in that position for six to eight seconds as shown in Fig. 26.

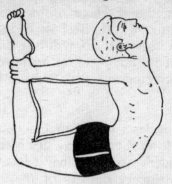

Fig. 26 *Ushtra asana.*

(iv) After holding for the desired seconds return to the position of readiness with the following process:

Release the left hand first and straighten up the left side of the body a little. Then release the right hand and make the body straight. If possible, sit on the soles and in between the heels and then rest. You have completed one round of *Ushtra asana.*

(v) After resting for six to eight seconds repeat the process a few more times.

Daily Practice: Do it only twice daily during the first week. During the second week and afterwards repeat it a maximum of four times daily.

Benefits: For the asthmatics *Ushtra asana* brings a beneficial effect upon the whole of the respiratory system. This *asana* activates the facial tissues, the nasal passage, the pharynx, the lungs and the whole of the respiratory organs and the nerves. Because of internal as well as external stimulation during this *asana*, the weakened condition of the organs of respiration is corrected and their normal health is restored.

Ushtra asana has several beneficial effects for everyone. It alleviates many disorders of the neck, shoulders, and the spine. It cures various types of visionary defects of the eyes and strengthens all the sense organs. People suffering from throat trouble, tonsil, voice defect and chronic headache will find this *asana* very beneficial. It also has a beneficial effect upon the muscles of the chest and helps in making the chest area proportionate in size. It is not a difficult *asana*. With a little practice any person can do it.

SIMHASANA
Position of Readiness: Put a blanket or a towel on the floor. Kneel on the floor with the hips and buttocks resting in the curve of the soles and the heels. If this proves to be difficult sit in the position nearest this which is the most comfortable.

Make the body straight. Keep the head, the neck and the spine in one line. Look straight ahead. Place the palms face down on the knees. Breathe normally. This is the position of readiness for *Simhasana*.

Steps of Actual Practice: *(i)* Start exhaling partially through both nostrils and partially through the mouth and at the same time start extending out the tongue. Do not rush. Gradually let the tongue come as far out of the mouth as possible. By the time the tongue has been pushed out, the exhalation should be over. Then hold the breath.

(ii) When the tongue is fully out do the following steps. Spread out the fingers of both hands and tighten them. Open the eyes wide and make them look frightening. Keep the whole body tense. Stay in this tense and strained condition for about six to eight seconds. You are in the *Simhasana* as shown in Fig. 27.

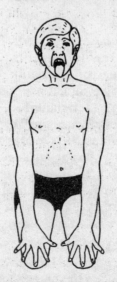

Fig. 27 *Simhasana*.

(iii) After holding the *asana* for a few seconds, start inhaling and withdrawing the tongue. Let the body be gradually loosened while inhaling and pulling back the tongue. When the tongue has been fully withdrawn, close the mouth and breathe normally and rest for a few seconds. Let the whole body be relaxed, while sitting in the same position.

(iv) After resting for six to eight seconds repeat the process a few more times.

Daily Practice: Begin with two rounds daily during the first week. From the second week onward make four rounds daily. Do not make more than four rounds in a single sitting. In certain cases this *asana* can be performed twice daily after giving a gap of eight hours between the first and the second sitting.

Benefits: *Simhasana* is very famous for its various remarkable benefits. It has some medicinal value for alleviating throat trouble, loss of the voice and tonsillitis.

It also has a beneficial effect on the respiratory system. It activates the larynx, trachea and all the bronchioles. It provides an invigorating effect on the thyroid cartileges. Because of these internal activations and invigorations, there is some restoration of health to the whole of the respiratory system and its disorder is removed. This is an easy *asana*.

SARVANGASANA

Position of Readiness: Lie down on your back on the floor. Keep the palms down and near to the body. Bring the heels and toes together and keep them relaxed. Make the whole body straight and look towards the ceiling. Breathe normally. This is the position of readiness.

Steps of Actual Practice: *(i)*Stretch out the toes of both legs and make them tense. Then start inhaling and at the same time start lifting both legs together towards the ceiling. Inhale slowly so that by the time the legs have been brought to a perpendicular position, inhaling is completed.

(ii) Just as the inhaling is completed and both the legs have been brought fully upward, bring both the palms under the hip, and raise the whole body upward by pushing it with both hands while exhaling.

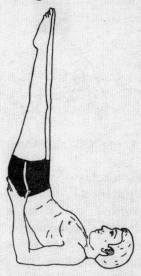

Fig. 28 *Half Sarvangasana.*

Do not try to raise the body with any excessive strain. Go only as high as your body permits (see Fig. 28). Keep both the palms on each side of the back for support. When the body has been raised to a maximum point (as shown in Fig. 29), stay there and breathe normally.

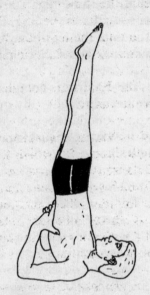

Fig. 29 *Sarvangasana.*

Tense the muscles of the legs and keep them together. Stay in this position for ten to fifteen seconds during the first week. Gradually increase the time to one minute a month and up to three minutes during the second month.

(iii) After standing on the shoulders for the desired seconds or minutes, return to the ground according to the following method:

Bend the legs first. This will bring the heels near the hips. Now gradually move the palms towards the hips and let the body come down slowly to the floor. While returning, support the body's weight with the hands. Make it a smooth return. When the hips touch the ground, drop the heels nearer the hips first. Put the palms on the floor on both sides of the body. Then stretch out the legs and let them fall on the floor. You have made one round of *Sarvangasana*. Now rest.

(iv) Rest for about ten seconds. During the rest breathe as normal.

Daily Practice: Sarvangasana is done only once. But the length of time for which the position is held can be increased. Those who have practised this *asana* for more than a month can hold it for three minutes. The maximum time for holding it is three minutes. The beginners should start it with ten seconds only and should increase the time gradually.

Benefits: Sarvangasana is one of the most valued *asana* of the Hatha Yoga system. As its name indicates it is indeed an *asana* of the whole body. There is hardly any area of the body which is not energized, activated and exercised during this *asana*. Because of its completeness in its effect, it is regarded next only to the king of all *asana* – *Sirshasana*.

For the asthmatics, *Sarvangasana* has medicinal value. It exercises all the bronchioles and the whole of the lungs. It removes the weakening condition of the lungs through internal activation. Since the whole of the respiratory system is invigorated and strengthened during this *asana*, the troubles of the lungs are corrected.

This *asana* has countless beneficial effects. Therefore it is a very desirable *asana* for everybody. It corrects any disorder of the circulatory system, supplies blood to the facial tissues, removes constipation, gastric disorders, and abdominal troubles, strengthens the digestive system and energizes the thyroid and all the sex glands. It is good for both males and females.

MATSYASANA

The method of practising *Sarvangasana* has been described in the preceding pages. After practising *Sarvangasana* it is necessary to practise *Matsyasana*. This is for a very good reason. Certain *asanas* activate certain parts of the body more than the others. In order to balance this out some *asanas* are followed by certain other *asanas*. For example, during *Sarvangasana* the head, the neck and the shoulders become passive and the lower areas of the body become active. In order to create a balance, it is followed by *Matsyasana* so that the head, the neck and the shoulders become active and the lower areas of the body remain passive. Thus by doing the *Matsyasana* after the *Sarvangasana*, activation of the whole body is completed in a balanced way.

There are two ways of doing the *Matsyasana*:- With or without the Lotus pose.

Though the first form is regarded as superior to the second; basically both are equally beneficial. Since it is not possible for everyone to take up the Lotus position both forms are described so that every person can practise it.

Position of Readiness: Make any one of the following two positions:

(i) Lie on the back with the legs crossed in the Lotus form. After allowing the spine, neck and head to fall on the floor, completely let the thighs also fall down. Put the hands on the floor near to the body. Keep the palms facing down. Breathe normally. This is the position of readiness using the Lotus position. If you cannot do this, try the second method as described below:

(ii) Lie on the floor on your back. Bend the legs and bring the heels near the hips. Keep the knees together and the heels about four inches apart. Put the palms on the floor. Make the body straight. Look upward and breathe normally. This is the easy starting position.

Steps of Actual Practice: Bring the palms under the thighs. While giving a pull on the thighs lift the head slightly upward. Let the weight of the upper area of the body rest on the elbows. Then bend the head backward and make an arch form by bending the backbone. When the arch form is made, rest the head on the floor. To produce a bigger arch give more pull on the thighs and more twist on the neck and back. But don't overdo it. In the beginning start with a minimum pull.

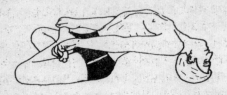

Fig. 30 *Matsyasana in Lotus Pose.*

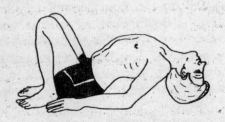

Fig. 31 *Easy Matsyasana.*

(ii) When the arch has been made according to the suitability of your body, stay there in that form. If you are in the Lotus position, then hold the toes of the left leg with the right hand and those of the right leg with the left hand and lightly pull them as shown in Fig. 30. If you are doing the *Matsyasana* the easy way, stretch out the hands on the side of the body and keep the palms on the floor as shown in Fig. 31.

(iii) Now make a few deep but slow and gradual breaths. Stay in this position for about six to eight seconds. This makes the *Matsyasana* completely done.

(iv) After being in *Matsyasana* for the desired period return to the position of readiness with the following process: In case you were holding the toes, leave them and bring the palms down on the floor. Then pull the thighs with your hands again by bending the arms. Now lift the head upwards and strengthen the neck and head. Then gradually bring the back, shoulders, neck and head to the floor, unfold the legs and stretch them on the floor and rest.

(v) Rest for two to three normal breaths. After the rest is over, repeat the process two or three times.

Daily Practice: For asthmatics, *Matsyasana* has several beneficial effects. It corrects disorders of the respiratory system as a whole. This is because all the organs concerned with respiration, such as the nasal passage, the pharynx, the larynx, the trachea, the bronchi and the lungs are well exercised during this *asana*. *Matsyasana* provides several other benefits. It has a beneficial effect on the facial tissues. It activates the spine and all the muscles of the back. As a result of this activation disorders of the spine and back can be alleviated. It removes stiffness of the neck and back and brings flexibility to the whole upper area of the body. It has a good effect upon their malfunctioning.

Its easy form can be practised by any person of any age group. Since it is a highly beneficial *asana*, it is recommended to everyone.

5.

Arthritis

Arthritis is a disease of the joints. The people suffering from this disease have a burning feeling, terrible pain and aching in their affected joints. There is swelling, redness, stiffness, and heat in the joints. There are several variations of arthritis. The most common types are the rheumatoid arthritis, and osteoarthritis.

It is difficult to explain the root cause of all these kinds of arthritis as there are various reasons for it. For example, it could be due to lack of proper diet, lack of proper exercise, lack of hygienic care, and similar other factors.

All over the world millions of people suffer from this vexing, tortuous and disabling disease. It affects both male and female of all age groups. The most disheartening aspect of the disease is that it is difficult to get rid of through medicine when it is in its chronic stage.

It is a common practice all over the world to give medicines and recommend physical exercises to the patients for treating this disease. Since therapeutic yoga is not yet well known to the orthodox medical practitioners they do not make use of it to treat arthritis.

In treating the patients of arthritis at our institute we have found that a regular practice of some selected yoga asanas may alleviate this disease within two months when it is in the early stages. In chronic cases it takes four to five months or even more to restore the sufferer to normal health. The most remarkable aspect of yoga treatment is that it treats the disease without the use of any medicine and the effects are usually permanent. Let me now explain the Yoga system of treatment.

Treatment

The arthritic or rheumatic patients have to do three things: *(i)* regular practice of selected yoga asanas, *(ii)* to eat a proper diet *(iii)* to maintain proper hygienic care. A detailed description of these aspects are explained below:

(i) Yoga Asana: The arthritics are advised to practice *Santulan Asana*, *Trikonasana*, *Veerasana*, *Gomukhasana*, *Briksha Asana*, *Setubandh Asana*, *Siddhasana*, *Natraj Asana*, and *Shava Asana*. The method of practising these *asanas* is presented one by one in the following pages. A regular practice of these *asanas* should alleviate arthritis of any type without the use of any medicine. Those who are used to taking medicine might be able to stop after they have practised yoga for two to three weeks.

(ii) Proper Diet: A proper diet for anyone means: to take what is beneficial and stop what

is harmful. Arthritic or rheumatic people are advised to stop taking the following things: banana, and curd (yogurt). Those who smoke and take tobacco in any form, should stop it completely or should reduce its intake considerably. No more than two cups of coffee or tea should be taken a day.

They should eat four times daily. For breakfast they should eat an orange, apple or any fruit (except banana), germinated gram, wheat bread and green vegetables. They can take a cup of hot milk with ovaltine. The non-vegetarians can take a boiled or poached egg. For lunch and dinner they should have a salad (a mixture of tomato, carrot, cucumber, radish, lettuce or any raw vegetables) followed by wheat bread, green vegetables, pulses . The non-vegetarians can eat fish and liver with the least amount of spices. They should avoid any excessive use of hot spices, should drink ten to twelve glasses of fresh water, and should eat at least two hours before going to bed.

In the afternoon, they should take some light refreshment, such as some fresh fruits, salted biscuits, cake or other similar items.

(iii) Hygienic Care: The most important thing about hygienic care is to take a regular bath, keep the whole body clean and take proper care of teeth. Bath can be taken with hot or cold water as desired. The whole body should be thoroughly rubbed with soap and a flannel in order to acheive the full benefit.

It is also important to wear clean clothes and underwear at all times. Neatness and cleanliness should be maintained in every day life as much as possible.

If the arthritics follow the above mentioned system of yoga therapy they should feel assured of obtaining some relief from this disease. They are advised to begin their practice according to the method described in this chapter. During the first week they should practise only two to four *asanas* of this series. During the second week and after they should gradually add other *asanas*. They should never try to do all the *asanas* of this series during the first week.

SANTULANASANA

Position of Readiness: Put a carpet or blanket or mat on the floor. Stand on the floor with the body straight and firm. Look straight ahead. Let the hands hang at the sides. This is the position of readiness.

Note: In order to do this asana you will have to stand on one leg at a time. It is not easy for everyone to stand on one leg. Therefore, those who might have any difficulty in standing on one leg, should stand near a pillar or the wall for supporting the body weight.

Steps of Actual Practice: (i) Stand up on the right leg and bend the left leg. Bring the heel of the left leg near the hip. If the heel cannot be brought nearer the hip due to pain in the knee, fold the leg backward, as much as possible.

(ii) Catch the toes of the left leg with the left hand in such a way that all the toes are held with the palm. Bring the heel of the bent leg to the hip or nearer to it.

(iii) Tense the right hand. Keep all the fingers together and slowly raise the right hand up towards the sky. Do not rush in lifting the hand. Keep the palm facing downwards, while raising the hand. When the hand is fully raised the palm should remain in the straight forward position.

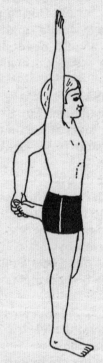

Fig. 32 *Santulanasana.*

(iv) Stay in that position for six to eight seconds. Keep the lifted hand tense. The right

leg on which you are standing should be tight and straight. Keep looking straight ahead. There is no special breathing requirement in this *asana*. Keep breathing in normally, while doing this *asana*.

(v) After staying in this position for six to eight seconds, return to the position of readiness by the following process. Slowly bring the lifted hand down, keeping it tensed. Do not drop the hand. When the raised hand has reached the side, release the left leg to come on the floor. You are now in the position of readiness again after completing one round of *Santulanasana*.

After resting for six seconds stand on the left leg and bend the right leg and raise the left hand in the same way as you did the first time. Make further rounds alternately by following the same process.

Daily Practice: Do it only four times daily during the first week. After practising for a week, increase to six times a day.

Benefits: *Santulanasana* is mainly a *kriya* of the major joints of the body. It removes rigidity and brings flexibility to them. It also normalizes the blood circulation in the affected areas and tones up the muscles. As a result of enhanced blood circulation, flexibility and muscle conditioning, pain in the joints is corrected.

This *asana* has a beneficial effect upon disorders of the knees, ankles, shoulder joints, wrists, palms and fingers. It is an easy *asana* and any person can practise it either standing on the floor or with the help of the wall. It is a good *asana* for body activation and flexibility in the joints.

TRIKONASANA

Position of Readiness: Stand with the legs about two and half feet apart. Look straight ahead. Let the hands hang loosely on the sides. Make the legs firm and tight.

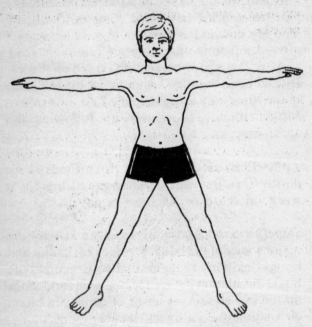

Fig. 33 *First Phase of Trikonasana.*

Steps of Actual Practice: (i) Inhale slowly and at the same time raise both the hands up to the level of the shoulders. Keep the hands tense while raising them up. This will bring both hands in one line. The palms should be facing downwards. By the time the hands have come up in one line, inhaling should be completed. Stay there for two seconds. You should be as shown in Fig. 33.

(ii) Then start exhaling and simultaneously lower the left hand to touch the left foot and raise the right hand. By the time you have touched the foot you should have completed exhaling. When exhaling is over hold the breath.

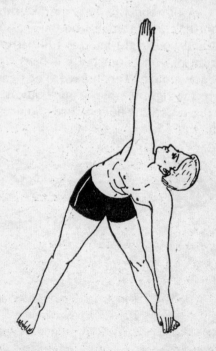

Fig. 34 *Second Phase of Trikonasana.*

While going down bend forward, not sideways. Keep looking at the toes you are going to touch. Try to touch the toes of the left foot. After touching the toes, turn your head to the right and raise it towards the sky. Now try to see the palm of the right hand. At this point your hands are again in one line. Keep looking at the right palm for about two seconds. Do not bend your legs. Keep the leg muscles tensed up (see Fig. 34 for this second phase).

(iii) After looking at the right palm for a few seconds bring the upper hand in front and then look on the floor beneath that palm. During this stage your left hand remains on the toes of the left foot and your right hand is fully stretched out in front of you. Your body is bent right in front. Legs should be kept tensed. The right arm is close to the right temple. You should still be holding the breath. Your posture should be as shown in Fig. 35.

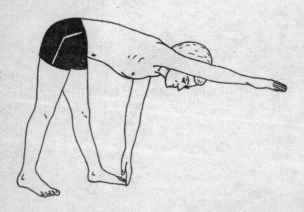

Fig. 35 *Third Phase of Trikonasana*

(iv) Then move the right hand by forty-five degrees to the right side while keeping the arm and the hand quite stretched. At this stage the fingers of the right hand are together and the palm is about one foot above the ground. Look at the ground where the fingers of the right hand are pointing as shown in Fig. 36. Stay in this position for two seconds. Keep holding the breath.

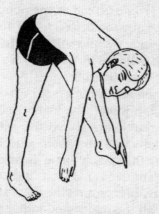

Fig. 36 *Final Phase of Trikonasana.*

Now bring the right hand to the right leg and start inhaling and standing up. While standing up, allow your hands to drag lightly on the legs till you are back in the standing position. After returning to the position of readiness your hands are again at the side. You have completed one round of *Trikonasana*. Now rest for two normal breaths.

(v) After resting for about five seconds repeat the *asana* by following the same process. In the

second round you have to touch the right foot and raise the left hand towards the sky. Repeat the process a few times.

Daily Practice: Make four alternate rounds daily during the first week. During the second week and afterwards make six rounds daily. Never make more than eight rounds in a single day.

Benefits: *Trikonasana* has medicinal value for alleviating pains or disorders of the neck and shoulder joints. People suffering from stiffness in the neck will find this *asana* very effective in correcting that disorder.

This *asana* has a beneficial effect upon the spine, the hip joints, the hands and the palms. All the major joints above the waist area are properly activated and their muscles are duly toned up by this *asana*. Arthritics are advised to practise *Santulanasana* first and then the *Trikonasana* by performing the exercises one after the other, all the major and minor joints of the body are activated and their functioning is normalized.

Trikonasana has beneficial effects for everyone. It develops the visionary power of the eyes; brings flexibility to the spine; and improves concentration. It is an easy *asana* and hence recommended to everyone.

VEERA ASANA
Position of Readiness: Be seated on the floor in a relaxed way. Keep the body straight. Look straight ahead. Breathe normally.

Steps of Actual Practice: *(i)* Bend one leg behind you so the hips are resting on its heel. The toes of this leg should fall on the ground. The heel is up, touching the hip. There is no body weight on the folded leg, all the weight of the body is on the floor.

(ii) Bend the other leg and place it across the thigh of the leg you are kneeling on, allowing the knee to rest on the floor. (See Fig 37)

(iii) Stretch both hands out to the sides and then bring the wrists on the head. Then join the palms and the fingers of both hands close together. Keep the wrists on the top of the head and keep the fingers pointing straight upwardly.

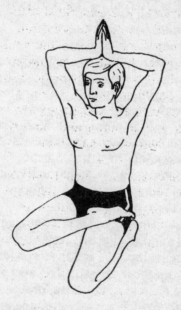

Fig. 37 *Veera asana*

Then try to straighten the elbows as much as is comfortably possible.

(iv) Now straighten the spine, the neck and the head. Look in front. Keep the palms and the fingers together. Your elbows should remain straight and tight. Keep breathing in a normal way. You are in *Veera asana.* Stay in this position for eight seconds.

(v) After eight seconds, unfold the palms and bring down the hands. Then lift the upper foot by hand and bring it down on the floor. Then pull back the other folded leg and bring it to an easy pose. Now rest for five seconds. You have completed one round of *Veera asana.* Repeat the process alternating the positions with each leg.

Daily Practice: Do four rounds daily. It may be increased to a maximum of six rounds. Do not practise more than six rounds in a single day.

Benefits: *Veera asana* exercises all the major and minor joints in a single process in a very effective way. The external activation enhances the blood circulation in the joint areas and restores their normal health.

The *asana* has also a strengthening effect on the lungs and the chest. It tones up the muscles of the thighs, the hips and the arms and reduces the fat from these areas. It has also a symbolic value. It is held that those practising *Veera asana* will develop courage, boldness and bravery.

GOMUKHASANA

Position of Readiness : The proper position of readiness of *Gomukhasana* might be difficult to make for those arthritics whose knees, ankles and toes are severely affected. Therefore, such patients are advised to sit on the floor by simply bending the knees and keeping the spine straight upwardly.

Those who can make the proper position of readiness should sit on the floor according to the following steps: Kneel on the floor ensuring that the weight is evenly distributed. Keep the knees about four inches apart. Let the ankles and toes of both the legs fall on the floor in such a way that the toes are brought close to one another but the heels are upwards, spread out.

This will make an arch-like curve with the toes, soles and the heels. Then gradually sit down on the curve of the soles, putting the whole weight of the body on it. Put the palms on the thigh. Look straight ahead. Keep the spine quite straight. You are now in the perfect position of readiness for *Gomukhasana* as shown in Fig. 15.

Steps of Actual Practice: *(i)* Slowly bring the right hand to the back. Bend it at the right elbow and then raise the back of the palm up towards the neck. This will keep the back of the palm pressed against the spine. Let the fingers of the right hand face upwards. Keep the right hand firmly in that position.

(ii) Bend your left arm and raise it upwards by

putting the left palm on the left shoulder. Then, first try to touch the fingers of the left hand with the right hand. Some people might have difficulty in even touching the fingers. They should try to get them as near as possible and then stay there. Those who do not have any difficulty in touching the fingers should make a lock by folding the fingers of both the hands. For making the lock the fingers are slightly crooked and then these crooks may be hooked together and pulled against each other.

(iii) After making the lock with the fingers of both hands, try to raise the elbow of the left hand straight upwards. Keep the spine firm and straight. Look in front. Breathe normally. Stay in this locked position for six to eight seconds. Those who cannot make the lock should

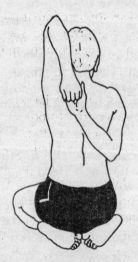

Fig. 38 *Gomukhasana.*

attempt to attain this position as much as is possible and then should stay there for six to eight seconds in the same position. When the fingers of one hand are locked against the fingers of the other hand in that sitting position it completes the *Gomukhasana* as shown in Fig. 38.

(iv) After staying in that position for six to eight seconds, loosen the grip on the fingers and then unlock the fingers gradually. Then slowly bring both the hands on the thighs and rest. You have made one round of *Gomukhasana*. After resting for two normal breaths make more rounds alternately by following the same process. That means you have to bring now the left hand across the back and raise the elbow of the right hand.

Daily Practice: Repeat four times daily during the first week. During the second week and afterwards make six rounds daily. Do it alternately.

Benefits: *Gomukhasana* has, as a single exercise, a corrective effect upon all the major and minor joints of the body. It exercises the finger joints, the elbows, the shoulder joints, the toes, the ankles, the knees and the hip joints very effectively. All the muscles and nerves related to various joints are automatically toned up, activated and normalized.

Because of activation of the muscles of the joints, blood circulation is improved in these areas. As a result, the waste products are removed from the joints. It restores the synovial fluid (joint fluid) and thereby enables easier movement and alleviates pain

This asana has many beneficial effects for everyone. It brings flexibility to the joints, strengthens the bones, increases the measurement of the chest, and increases the strength of the lungs and heart.

VRIKSHASANA

Postion of Readiness: Stand up on the floor. Look straight ahead. Keep the hands hanging loose at the sides. Make the body straight and firm. Breathe normally. This is the position of readiness.

Steps of Actual Practice: You have to stand up on one leg for practising this *asana*. In case you have difficulty in standing on one leg, use a wall or a pillar for support. Then do the following steps:

(i) Stand on the left leg and bend the right leg at the knee. Bring the right foot to the thigh of the left leg so that the outer part of the heel and sole rest on the left thigh. This will twist the right foot a little and press its side against the left thigh. Do not press the thigh with the heel itself but with its side. When the side of the heel has been firmly pressed against the left thigh, make the left leg and the whole body erect and straight.

(ii) Then raise both hands sideways towards the head. When the hands are stretched above the head join the palms and the fingers together.

Then bring the palms on the head so that the wrists rest on the head.

(iii) When the palms have been joined above the head, try to give a backward pull on the folded elbows in order to bring them in one line. But do not exert too much. Look straight ahead Tighten the leg you are standing on. The whole body should be tensed. You should be breathing normally. Stay in that position for six to eight seconds. You are in *Vrikshasana* as shown in Fig. 39.

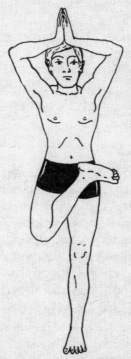

Fig. 39 *Vrikshasana.*

(iv) After holding that *asana* for the desired period, loosen the pressure on the palms and stretch out the arms in order to bring them back to their original position. When the hands are in position, hold the toes of the folded leg, lift it slightly upwards and then drop it on the floor. you are now back in the position of readiness. Rest for two normal breaths.

(v) After resting for a few seconds, repeat the *asana* a few more times, alternating with leg positions.

Daily Practice: Make four rounds daily during the first week. During the second week and afterwards make six rounds daily. Keep alternating the leg position while repeating the exercise. Do not practise it more than six rounds in a single day.

Benefits: *Vrikshasana* activates all the joints of the body. All the major and minor joints of the body are affected by this single *asana*. It tones up the muscle of the ankles, toes, knees, hip joints, shoulder joints, elbows, hands and fingers. As a result of activation and conditioning of the joint muscles, blood circulation becomes normal in the joints and they regain strength.

For everyone *Vrikshasana* has beneficial effects upon their bodily joints and bones. It brings flexibility to the legs and hands and enhances the measurement of the chest. It is an easy *asana* and hence everyone can do it.

SEDHUBANDHASANA

Position of Readiness: Lie down on your back
on the floor. Bend the legs and bring the heels
nearer the hip. Keep the heels and the knees
about two to three inches apart. Bring your
hands close to the body on both sides. Put the
palms on the floor. Look straight up. Breathe
normally. This is the position of readiness.

Steps of Actual Practice: *(i)* Lift the hips and the
waist upwards while keeping the shoulders and
the feet on the floor. When the hips have been
raised upwards, support them with both
hands

(ii) Gradually keep raising the hips upwards
while pushing the palms towards the waist area.
Let the hands help raising the waist upwards as
high as it can be raised without strain. Now
support the body weight on the thumbs and the
index fingers. Let the shoulders, neck and the
head be firmly on the floor. Try to check that
the thighs are parallel to one another with about
a gap between of three inches. Keep breathing
normally. Stay in this position for six to eight
seconds.

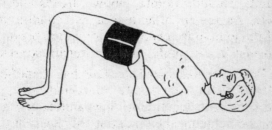

Fig. 40 *Sedhubandasana*

(iii) After remaining in the raised up position for six to eight seconds, start lowering the hips towards the floor while still supporting the body weight on the palms, do not let the body drop on the floor, bring it down slowly. When the hips, the waist and the back are on the floor put your palms on the floor on both sides of the body. Stretch out the legs on the floor and rest for two to three normal breaths.

(iv) After resting for a few seconds repeat the *asana* by following the same process.

Daily Practice: Make four rounds daily during the first week. During the second week and afterwards make a maximum of six rounds. Do not ever attempt more than six rounds in a single day.

Benefits: The main impact of *Sedhubandhasana* is on the spine and the hip joints. Those who have pain either in any part of the spine or in the hip joints are strongly advised to practise this *asana*. This *asana* also relieves pain and corrects disorders of the shoulder joints, neck, arms and the palms. Since it is an easy *asana*, arthritics in any condition and of any age can practise it.

It is a good *asana* for creating flexibility in the spine, for removing wind and gastric troubles, and for correcting respiratory disorders.

SIDHASANA
Persons with moderate joint pain of any type can be helped if they practise the *asana* of this series already described above. The chronic

cases, however, might take a little longer time for getting complete recovery. Therefore, the arthritis patients with chronic trouble are advised to keep practising all the *asanas* of this series regularly. By continuing the practice they should be recovering in two to three months.

It needs to be emphasized that one must eat a proper diet along with the regular practice of yoga in order to get a satisfactory result. The diet for the arthritics has been fully described in the first part of this chapter. It is expected that the arthritics take their meals according to those recommendations. I wish only to remind them not to take curd, banana, and to avoid taking tea and smoking cigarettes on an empty stomach. With these clarifications, a new *asana* – *Sidhasana* – is presented now. The method of practice and its benefits are described below:

Position of Readiness: Be seated on the carpeted floor. Stretch out both the legs in front. Keep your spine straight. Look straight ahead. Keep the hands down on the floor. Breathe normally. This is the position of readiness.

Steps of Actual Practice: (i) Bend the left leg back from the knee and bring the foot in front. Then stretch the toes and ankle of the left leg and try to bring them in a straight line. In case you find it difficult to bring them in a straight line, stretch them out as far as possible. Now your left knee should be on the floor. In case the knee cannot touch the floor, let it remain a little up and raised.

(ii) Now bend the right leg and bring the right foot on the top of the left foot. Keep the right heel just above the left heel. Then stretch the toes and ankle of the right leg while keeping the right knee also on the floor. Keep the legs in the same position.

(iii) Stretch out both the hands. Make a circular shape with your thumb and the index finger in each hand. Then stretch out the remaining three fingers of each hand and keep them firmly together. Now put the right wrist on the right knee and the left wrist on the left knee. Tense the arms and the hands. Keep the spine straight and firm.

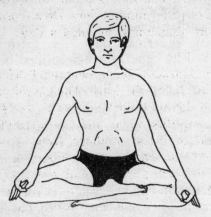

Fig. 41 *Sidhasana.*

Your head, neck and the spine should be in one line. Your fingers should be pointing towards the ground. Keep looking straight ahead. Breathe normally. Now you are in *Sidhasana*, as shown in Fig. 41.

(iv) Stay in this position for about one minute, then loosen the fingers of both the hands. Then lift up the right leg by hand and put it down on the floor and stretch out the legs. Rest for a few seconds and alternate the position of the legs. This time your right foot will be underneath and the left foot will be on the top. Stay in this *asana* again for about a minute.

Daily Practice: Practice *Sidhasana* for a maximum of three minutes only. Begin with about two minutes and gradually increase the time to three minutes daily. During this period you will be doing *Sidhasana* only twice and the total time spent will be three minutes only. Do not practise it for more than three minutes a day.

Benefits: *Sidhasana* has a beneficial effect on all the joints below the waist. The hip joints, the knees and the ankles are very effectively activated during this *asana* and, as a result, the circulation of blood in these areas becomes normalized, the supply of synovial fluid (joint fluid) is restored, and immobility and pain are removed. *Sidhasana* has a good effect on the nervous system all over the body. People suffering from any kind of nerve defects will find this *asana* very beneficial. It is regarded as a vitally important *asana* for gaining power of concentration and for acquiring mental balance. Though it might appear a little difficult *asana* for the beginners, with regular practice, any person can do it properly.

NATARAJASANA

Position of Readiness: Stand on the floor. Let the hands hang loosely on the sides. Make the body firm and straight. Look straight ahead. Breathe normally. This is the position of readiness.

Steps of Actual Practice: *(i)* Stand up on the left leg. Bend the right leg behind you and hold the toes with the right hand. At this stage your right leg is just folded backwards and it is held by the palm. Keep the leg in the same position.

(ii) Then bring all the fingers of the left hand together and tense the left hand. When the left hand has been tightened, slowly raise this hand up and at the same time slowly push the right leg backwards. In this process you are doing two things simultaneously. You are raising the left hand in front and pushing the right foot backwards. While doing this, you should give a backwards push with the right leg. But do not raise the left hand straight up towards the sky, keep it slanting, pointed towards the horizon, so that the whole hand is visible to you.

(iii) Now bend the body above the waist slightly forward and try to see the top of the fingers of the left hand and keep looking there. Keep the right foot fully pushed back. Make the left leg quite firm. Do not loosen the left leg when you bend the body slightly forward. Stay in this position for about eight seconds. Keep breathing normally, all through this *asana*. In case you have difficulty in doing this *asana* on the floor, stand with the support of either a wall

or a pillar. After you have become used to practising it, do it standing on the floor, without any support.

(iv) After remaining in this position for about eight seconds, gradually bring the left hand

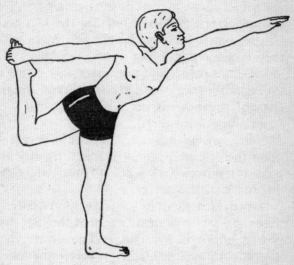

Fig. 42 *Natarajasana*

down and bring the right leg back to the folded position and then release it. You are now standing on both legs. Rest in that position for a while. After resting for a few seconds, repeat the *asana*. This time stand up on the right leg, hold the left leg and raise the right hand. Repeat the process alternating the position of the leg each time.

Daily Practice: Make four rounds daily during the first week. During the second week and afterwards make six rounds daily. Do not make more than six rounds of *Natarajasana* in a single day.

Benefits: *Natarajasana* activates all the major and minor joints of the body in a single process. For the arthritics it has a beneficial effect upon all the joints. It brings proper activation upon the shoulder joints, hip joints, the knees, the ankles, the palms and the fingers. Because of this conditioning, the muscles, nerves and tissues of these areas get normalized and their functioning is restored.

Natarajasana has also a beneficial effect upon the spine. It removes spinal rigidity and pain. It removes back ache, stiffness, and other disorders of the spine.

It provides flexibility to the limbs, strengthens the major bones, enhances the digestive power, improves eyesight, and generates vitality, potency and the quality of determination. A significant aspect of *Natarajasana* is that it symbolizes action. In other words it breaks the condition of immobility in the individual and creates a feeling to act. Because of these benefits, it is a highly recommended *asana* for the arthritics as well as for other practisers of yoga.

6.

Obesity

Obesity is now becoming a worldwide health hazard. Millions of people, male and female of every age, are carrying excessive extra weight on their bodies which they should not carry. The most frightening aspects of obesity are that it shortens the life span, causes atherosclerosis, coronary heart troubles, hypertension (high blood pressure), various physical-mental (psychosomatic) ailments and disorders, and makes the life of the person miserable due to development of such complications as gastrointestinal disorders, sexual incapacitation and the prospect of an inferiority complex. Let me explain in detail what it is, what are the causing factors, and how it is corrected through the yoga method.

For a better understanding of the problems related to obesity, we have to differentiate it from over-weight. Overweight is not obesity.

AVERAGE WEIGHT FOR MEN AND WOMEN

MEN

Weight in lbs. according to age

Feet	Inches	15 to 19 yrs	20 to 24 yrs	25 to 29 yrs	30 to 34 yrs	35 to 39 yrs	40 to 44 yrs	45 to 49 yrs	50 to 54 yrs	55 to 59 yrs
5	0	113	119	124	127	129	132	134	135	136
5	1	115	121	126	129	131	134	136	137	138
5	2	118	124	128	131	133	136	138	139	140
5	3	121	127	131	134	136	139	141	142	143
5	4	124	131	134	137	140	142	144	145	146
5	5	128	135	138	141	144	146	148	149	150
5	6	132	139	142	145	148	150	152	153	154
5	7	136	142	146	149	152	154	156	157	158
5	8	140	146	150	154	157	159	161	162	163
5	9	144	150	154	158	162	164	166	167	168
5	10	148	154	158	163	167	169	171	172	173
5	11	153	158	163	168	172	175	177	178	179
6	0	158	163	169	174	178	181	183	184	185
6	1	163	168	175	180	184	187	190	191	192
6	2	168	173	181	186	191	194	197	198	199

WOMEN

Weight in lbs. according to age

Feet	Inches	15 to 19 yrs	20 to 24 yrs	25 to 29 yrs	30 to 34 yrs	35 to 39 yrs	40 to 44 yrs	45 to 49 yrs	50 to 54 yrs	55 to 59 yrs
5	0	108	115	118	121	124	128	131	133	134
5	1	110	117	120	123	126	130	133	135	137
5	2	113	120	122	125	129	133	136	138	140
5	3	116	123	125	128	132	136	139	141	143
5	4	119	126	129	132	136	139	142	144	146
5	5	122	129	132	136	140	143	146	148	150
5	6	126	133	136	140	144	147	151	152	153
5	7	130	137	140	144	148	151	155	157	158
5	8	134	141	144	148	152	155	159	162	163
5	9	138	145	148	152	156	159	163	166	167
5	10	142	149	152	155	159	162	166	170	173
5	11	147	153	155	158	162	166	170	174	177
6	0	150	157	159	162	165	169	173	177	182

1 Kilo = 2.205 lbs.

But every obese person is overweight. Over-weight means carrying only a few pounds of extra weight than the body-frame requires. In case of overweight, though there is unwanted and extra weight, it may not be quite as excess-ive as obesity. For example, if a grown-up person of average height carries five to ten pounds of extra weight, he is overweight but not obese.

Unlike the overweight, the obese person's weight becomes almost static. Any adult person of average height who for a few years has been carrying more than ten pounds of extra weight is an obese person. The excessive weight begins to strain all the bodily organs of the obese person constantly and as a consequence he faces health hazards. The chart given on the following page shows how much average weight men and women should have.

Though obesity causes the same dispropor-tionate accumulation of fat in men and women, there is some variation in them. In women, fat generally accumulates on the hips and the thighs. In men, accumulation is mostly in the abdominal area. But in the course of time, in chronic cases of obesity this accumulation of fat and muscle covers the whole body. The fat then is not only localized but found all over the body.

Causes of Obesity
Though it is difficult to pinpoint the exact cause of obesity, it can fairly be stated that it is a consequence of excessive eating. It is true that

other factors are also involved in it, but one thing is certain that without excessive eating generally there will not be obesity.

In treating the patients of obesity at the Indian Institute of Yoga, Patna, and also at the Yoga Institute of Washington, D.C., U.S.A., I have found that all obese people develop certain common habits, make some common errors, and they all have the following common characteristics:

(i) They are addicted to over-eating,

(ii) They eat most of the time,

(iii) All of them, without exception, eat faster without chewing the food properly,

(iv) They retire soon after dinner,

(v) They either purposely avoid or do not get time to do physical labour and exercises.

We can say that obesity, as it prevails nowadays, is the result of modern civilization. All classes of people in the developed nations and the people of upper class in the developing nations are getting now more food and in many more varieties than it was possible centuries ago. Moreover, the scientific developments and modern facilities have made the life of the upper strata of the society so comfortable that they have hardly any need to do physical labour for a living. In the absence of any physical work, on the one hand, and daily intake of highly rich food, on the other, is bound to add extra weight.

Life today is now so highly mechanized that many people have hardly any physical labour to do at all. This combined with the increase in the amounts of rich, high-calorie foods available contributes to the overweight problem much of which is in the form of obesity. When the individual passes his days doing little but eating, he gets so much used to his routined life that he feels helpless and a victim of his own luxuries and comforts. Many become addicted to certain types of food and habits and they need treatment for restoration of normal health as any other patient of chronic disease would need.

Inferiority Complex

Another disheartening problem related to obesity is that the individual develops a feeling of inferiority. He does not like to meet his friends and the social groups. He begins to isolate himself and gets used to living a secluded life. In isolation or in company of his own type, he prefers to eat something most of the time and develops certain other bad habits, such as, taking alcoholic drinks, using intoxicating drugs and adopting various other harmful ways of living. The individual so isolated, develops various types of mental disorders, such as, nervousness, tension, anxiety, fear, lack of confidence, etc. Thus, he traps himself in a sort of a vicious circle. When he is nervous and anxious, he eats to pacify himself. And eating ultimately brings him back to the same mental condition he was already suffering from. Ultimately he develops various undesirable habits of living and it becomes difficult to restore him to normal health.

Yoga Method of Correcting Obesity
The Yoga method of correcting obesity primarily involves doing two things: *(i)* taking a balanced and proper diet, and *(ii)* practising a few selected *asanas*. Before describing how this is done, a few observations need to be made.

In treating sufferers from obesity at the Indian Institute of Yoga, Patna, and at the Yoga Institute of Washington, D.C., U.S.A., I have found that according to our process the average rate of reduction in weight is 1 to $1\frac{1}{2}$ lbs. per week which works out to about 4 to 6 pounds of weight per month. Depending upon his total extra weight, the correction period for an obese person lasts for some months. For example, if a person carries 42 pounds of extra weight, the correcting period might continue for seven to ten months.

The biggest advantage of this Yogic system of treament is that the individual does not have to go on fasting and he does not feel any weakness. The reduction in weight is so gradual that the person does not feel any loss of strength. Due to the gradual reduction, there is no sagging of the facial tissues or of the bodily skin and muscle. In this process, the reduction of weight and body conditioning occur simultaneously. As a result, by the time the sufferer has been restored to normal weight, his body becomes proportionate.

Manufactured Slimming Aids
It might be argued that the Yogic system takes too much time in correcting the excessive

weight, whereas several manufacturers and advertizers of weight-reducing gadgets, food packages, pills and drugs claim to reduce weight in a matter of days and weeks. Such advertisements probably attract millions of people by their big claims for reducing weight. But these 'gimmicks' do not bring any lasting result and cause various ailments, disorders and even do serious physical-mental harm to the users. I have been shocked to see several young girls and boys in the U.S.A. and also in India ruining their health, beauty and mental balance by using these 'gimmicks' and 'quickies'.

Advantages of the Yoga Method

The yoga method, though time-consuming, is preferable and desirable for several reasons. It reduces weight in a lasting and permanent way without causing any ill effect to health, beauty and physical-mental condition. It does not cost a penny to correct the disorder. There is no disturbance to normal life, nor is there any possibility of regaining the same weight if yoga practice is discontinued provided the same method of eating is maintained.

It is advised that once the weight has been reduced to normal level, the individual should keep practising yoga if only for ten to fifteen minutes per day. In case yoga practice is stopped for some reasons, the individual should continue to follow the yogic principles and method of eating. By taking a proper and balanced diet, the normality in weight will always remain the same. The overweight and obese persons are advised to eat according to the diet-chart given here.

DIET CHART FOR THE OBESE
Breakfast

i) Fruit juice – one cup of juice of any fruit, such as, orange, apple or pineapple.

ii) Fresh fruits – one apple, or banana, or two peaches.

iii) Sprouted gram(chickpeas) – $\frac{1}{4}$ cup

iv) Wheat bread or toast or muffins – two pieces, or cornflakes, or oatmeal with a little milk and sugar.

v) Egg – one (boiled, poached or scrambled).

vi) Tea or coffee – one cup.

Lunch and Dinner

i) Salad(a mixture of tomato, cucumber, radish, beets, celery, lettuce, carrot, etc., with salt, pepper and lemon juice or with salad dressing) – about one cupful.

ii) Soup of any type – one cupful.

iii) Rice, wheat bread or corn bread.

iv) Leafy vegetables of any kind.

v) Green vegetables of any kind.

vi) Pulses.

vii) Dessert: custard or fresh berries.

Note: The non-vegetarians can take fish liver or any sea-food, but should avoid taking other meats and chicken for a few months, if possible.

Snack

(i) Fresh fruit of any kind – one or two pieces
(ii) Salted biscuits – a few or nuts (a mixture of cashew, almond, pecan, pistachio and walnut) – $\frac{1}{4}$ cup
(iii) Tea or coffee – one cup (if needed)

The above-mentioned diet-chart provides just an outline of items to be taken for breakfast, lunch, tea-time and dinner. The chart does not explain the principles. Without observance of these vitally important aspects, just eating according to the diet-chart would not bring a satisfactory result. The chart becomes meaningful and important when the following principles, observed closely.

Points to Remember
(i) The first and most important principle is to eat slowly and chew and crush the food quite thoroughly.

(ii) The second vitally important principle is to finish eating at least two hours before going to sleep.

(iii) The third and the most important principle is: always eat a little less than you think you need to fill yourself.

(iv) Avoid drinking water while eating. Drink water half an hour after eating, Take ten to fifteen glasses of fresh water in twenty-four hours.

(v) Do not eat fatty, fried, and highly seasoned food. Avoid hot spices, pickles, *chutney* and sweets. Prepare your dishes by using the least amount of spices for flavour.

(vi) Eat only four times a day that is, take breakfast in the morning, lunch at noon, some light refreshment in the afternoon, and dinner at night. Avoid eating anything in between these four fixed hours.

By following the principles and method of eating as described above and by practising yoga *asana* as mentioned below, you can be sure of losing a minimum of six pounds a month.

Selected Yoga Asanas

The overweight and the obese have to practise yoga on a selected basis. It would not be possible for them to perform all types of *asanas* at the initial stage. Nor is it necessary to practise some of the difficult *asanas* for the desired result. There are several *asana* which are simple and easy to do, but have a remarkable effect on weight reduction and body-conditioning. Therefore, you are advised to begin your practise according to the selection of *asanas* given below:

A word of advice is that you should not try to do too many *asanas* in the beginning. Proceed gradually but regularly. Start with the *asanas* recommended for the first week and go on adding the *asanas* of the second, third and other weeks. This way your progress will be gradual, steady and without any strain and exhaustion. The result would begin to show right from the first week, even though you would be practising only a few yoga *asanas*.

First Week of Yoga Practice
During the first week, start with the following *asanas:*

1. *Ekpada Uttan asana* (as described in Chapter IV.) Make a total of eight rounds – four rounds with each leg alternately.
2. *Uttanpada asana* – (as described in Chapter II) Make a total of only four rounds daily. Never practise more than six rounds in a day.

Rest: After practising both the *asanas* noted above, rest in *Savasana* for a period of five minutes. See Chapter II for the method of practising *Savasana*

Second Week of Yoga Practice
Keep practising both the *asanas* of the first week and add the following *asanas*:

3. *Bhujangasana* – (as described in Chapter II) Practise four rounds daily.
4. *Salabhasana* – (as described in Chapter II) Practise four rounds daily.

After practising all the four *asanas*, rest in *Savasana* for five minutes.

Third Week of Yoga Practice
Keep practising all the four *asanas* of the preceding weeks and add the following *asanas* at the start of the third week:

5. *Santulanasana* – (as described in Chapter V) Make a total of six rounds daily – practise three rounds with each side, alternately.
6. *Pawanmuktasana* – (as described in Chapter II) Make a total of six rounds daily – practise three rounds with each side, alternately.

After practising all the six *asanas*, rest in savasana for a period of seven minutes.

Fourth Week of Yoga Practice
Keep practising all the six *asana* of the preceding weeks and add the following *asanas* at the beginning of fourth week:

7. *Suryanamaskar asana* – (as described in Chapter III) Make four rounds daily.
8. *Dhanurasana* – (as described in Chapter III) Make four rounds daily.

After practising all the eight *asanas*, rest in for a period of ten minutes

Fifth Week of Yoga Practice

Keep practising all the eight *asanas* of the preceding weeks and add the following *asanas* at the beginning of the fifth week:

9. *Ardhavakra asana* – (as described in Chapter III) Make only four rounds daily – two rounds with each side.
10. *Paschimottanasana* – (as described in Chapter II) Make only four rounds daily.

After practising all the *asanas*, rest now for ten minutes in *Savasana*

Sixth Week and Onwards

Add the following *asanas* during the sixth week and in your onward practice:

11. *Suptavajrasana* – (as described in Chapter III) Make only four rounds daily.
12. *Matseyendrasana* – (as described in Chapter III) Make only four rounds daily – two rounds with each side.

MANDUKASANA

Position of Readiness: For doing this *asana*, you need a padded floor. Therefore, put a blanket or folded cloth on the floor. Sit on your folded legs, as shown in Fig. 15. You should be in the same position as you have to be in the sitting position for making *Suptavajrasana*. Being seated in this position, breathe normally. This is the position of readiness.

Steps of Actual Practice: *(i)* Rest all your body weight on the right foot and lessen the weight on the left foot. This will make it possible for you to push the left foot out to the left side of the hip.

(ii) Then by putting all the body weight on the left side, release the right foot and push it out to the right side of the hip. Now you are sitting on the floor and your left foot is bent to the left side and the right foot is bent to the right side. Keep the palms on the floor to support the body weight. If this is painful do not proceed any further. Keep practising this far until there is no pain and then continue with the next stage.

(iii) While keeping hands on the floor on both sides and partially supporting the body weight, separate the knees gradually. Move the left knee further to the left side and right knee to the right side. Try to separate them as much as you can do so comfortably.

(iv) When the knees have been separated, stay there and do the following: Bring the palms on the knees on their respective side. Make the body straight. Look in front. Breathe normally. Stay in this position for eight to twelve seconds. You should be as shown in Fig. 43.

(v) After staying in that position for the desired time, return to the sitting position by the following method: Put your palms on the floor and make a kneeling position. Then bring forward any foot in front first by sliding it under

the hip area. Now bring the other leg also in front. Then sit comfortably and relax. After resting for six to eight seconds, repeat this *asana* a few times more by following the same process.

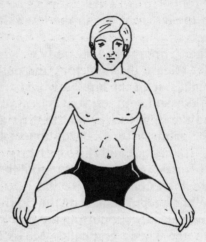

Fig. 43 *Mandukasana*

Daily Practice: Do it twice daily during the first week. Gradually develop the practice to a maximum of four times daily.

Benefits: It is a very effective *asana* for reducing fat around the thighs, hip and the abdominal areas. For both men and women, it has a beneficial effect on the muscles and nerves of the lower areas of the body.

This *asana* has several other benefits. It activates all the joints of the lower area of the body, enhances sexual potency, corrects disorders of the reproductive system, relieves piles, and strengthens the digestive system. With a little effort, this *asana* can be practised by any person.

7.

Mental Problems

The balance of the mind can become upset when an external or internal problem strains it harshly. Consequently, its functioning gets disturbed and its harmony begins to diminish, slowly or quickly depending upon the individual's state of mental health. The person so affected for a long period, becomes mentally sick with an intensity proportionate to the degree of harmony lost. As a result, the individual's thought, action, manner, behaviour and outlook becomes unbalanced, which takes various forms and shapes of abnormal expressions. This can involve persons of any age, background or race. Here, we are faced then, with two types of problems: *(i)* how to correct and cure the cases of mental sickness, and *(ii)* how and in what way one can maintain sound mental health. The answer to both — curative and preventive problems — we find in the system of yoga.

Causes of Mental Troubles

In order to understand the way in which Yoga can improve mental health, a brief discussion about the causes of mental troubles is essential. Most troubles which affect the mind of an individual spring from three basic sources: *(i)* nature, *(ii)* society, and *(iii)* self. In other words, the particular problem which strains and causes mental imbalance in an individual is either nature-oriented, society-oriented or self-oriented which have been termed at *Daivik, Bhautik* and *Atmik* by Kapil in his Samkhya philosophy.

The problems arising out of Nature could be in the form of some natural calamity, danger from certain animate creatures, and the peculiarity of natural phenomena. The societal problems, likewise, could be religious, ethnic, racial, economic, political, etc., or also they might involve the varied problems of adjustment to certain customs, manners, ways of life, etc., of a particular community. Similarly, there could be countless problems of the individual's own creation, which arise because of certain beliefs, faith, notions, habits, manners and also because of some inner feelings, such as, hatred, jealousy, revenge, love, romance, likes and dislikes.

People of every society, whether industrial, agrarian, tribal or primitive, have been faced with various problems arising out of these above-mentioned sources, more or less, in the same way as we have to face them today. Though the nature, forms and shapes of human problems have changed because of changes in social conditions, basically, they have remained the same. Seen in this context, it would be interesting to know what the early thinkers of yoga have thought over these human problems and what solutions they have provided.

Among the forefathers whose contribution became the foundation of yoga system one was called Kapil. Therefore, let us first see what Kapil had to say of this problem.

The contribution of Kapil(700 B.C.) is called Samkhya philosophy. According to Kapil, the answer to all human problems is in *Samyak jnana* (proper knowledge). In the absence of *samyak jnana*, the unfamiliar and peculiar happenings cause *dukha* (sorrow). When the individual develops and acquires proper knowledge about *Purusha* (self) and *Prakriti* (nature), then the undesirable results in any of the three sources mentioned above do not cause *dukha*. This implies acquiring a scientific knowledge about *rajas, tamas* and *sattva gunas,* and all the *tattvas* (elements) of *Prakriti* together with a knowledge about the composition, function and co-relationship of sense organs, action organs, mind, intelligence and the totality of the *urusha* (self). When the individual becomes so knowledgeable, he attains the power of overcoming pain, maintains mental balance and obtains pleasure and happiness.

But this Samkhya philosophy did not show the method and process of obtaining the goal. It needed a comprehensive system in order to help the individual adopt and achieve what had been so rightly stated by Kapil. This system was provided by Patanjali in his *Yoga Sutra*. Therefore, it is essential to understand what Patanjali had to say.

Patanajali's Yoga Sutra

The *Yoga Sutra* of Patanjali(300 B.C.) is a treatise on a simple process for obtaining the goal laid down by Kapil and adds something more. Whereas Kapil emphasized acquiring of *jnana* which involves only the mind, Patanjali's system of yoga on the other hand involves both mind and body. In this respect, the *Purusha* of Patanjali has to do two things simultaneously, that is, he must acquire *samyak jnana* and also he must perform yoga practices in order to achieve excellence of both body and mind. This way, by combining *jnana* and practices together the individual would attain not only excellent health but would also be able to maintain a harmonious relationship between the mind and the body. Thus, we find that Patanjali's yoga provides a better and more thorough answer to our problems of mental health than that which is provided by Kapil.

Since Patanjali's system involves knowing and doing both, his method includes all those steps which are essential for obtaining the desired goal on both levels — physical and mental. These steps are eight in number. They are mentioned below together with their basic meanings and implications: *Yama* (control and discipline), *Niyama* (rules, methods and principles), *Asanas* (making body postures), *Pranaya-*

ma (kriyas with air), *Pratyahara* (avoidance of taking undesirable actions, that is, knowing the proper action), *Dharana* (concentration), *Dhyana* (meditation), and *Samadhi* (contemplation).

Since these eight steps of Patanjali were not very comprehensively discussed in his *Yoga Sutra* further works were necessary for covering them properly. In order to facilitate the students of Yoga these steps were later grouped under different yogas according to their nature and substance. The yogas which cover all these steps are the following four:

JNANA YOGA covers *Yama* and *Niyama* and is the science of acquiring proper knowledge.

HATHA YOGA covers *Asana* and *Pranayamas* and is the science of physical excellence.

KARMA YOGA covers *Pratyahara* and is the science of action.

RAJA YOGA covers *Dharana*, *Dhyana*, and *Samadhi* and is the science of concentration and meditation.

Applied Yoga

It needs to be clearly stated here that not all types of mental cases can be helped through yoga. It is assumed that those going to practise yoga have the mental capability to understand its basic principles, methods and ideas and are physically in a condition to perform the simplest practices. Unless these basic requirements of the physical and mental conditions are fulfilled, it would be difficult to make proper use of yoga. With this understanding, the process of treatment and steps are described here. These recommendations are based on our experiences in correcting various cases of mental illness at the Indian Institute of Yoga, Patna.

Jnana and Karma Yogas

Persons suffering from mental disorders are advised to know the basic tenets of Jnana Yoga and Karma Yoga. Both these relate to the essentials of *samyak jnana* (acquiring of proper knowledge) and of *satkaryavad* (science of action). These yogas involve knowing certain basic concepts, theories, principles and thoughts concerning the self, society and nature. A knowledge of these would equip the individual to understand the causations and happenings in a given situation and would give him the knowledge to act properly for obtaining a satisfactory result. This being the importance of these two yogas, the individual should know them along with the practices of Hatha Yoga.

Guidelines

In order to achieve the fullest benefit of yoga it is important that the students have a proper understanding of the 'Essentials of Yoga Practice'. These essentials have been briefly described in Chapter 1. People with mental problems are advised to read the first chapter with special attention to: *(a)* therapeutic yoga, *(b)* essentials of yoga practice, *(c)* proper diet, and *(d)* bathing and cleaning. A proper understanding of these above-mentioned aspects and their adoption would provide a very satisfactory result to the students.

With the knowledge of the first chapter, they should begin practising Hatha Yoga according to the stages and steps outlined below:

Hatha Yoga

Hatha Yoga is comprised of *Pranayamas, asanas, bandhas* and *mudras*. People with mental problems are advised to practise only some of the selected items in the initial stage. When the normal mental condition is restored, they could try other items of Hatha Yoga according to their own liking and preference. With this understanding, they are recommended to begin their practice on the following basis:

First Week of Practice

They should begin with *Ujjayi Pranayama* in the 'lying position'. It is easy to do and any person can practise it. The method of practising *Ujjayi* in the 'lying position' is fully described in Chapter IV. They should practise only five rounds of it daily.

After making five rounds of Ujjayi, they should practise *Suryanamaskar asana* and *Uttanpadasana*. Four rounds of each of the above two *asana* would be sufficient. Do not make more than four rounds of each. Follow the method of doing *Suryanamaskar* as given in Chapter III and that of *Uttanpada* as given in Chapter II.

When all the three above-mentioned items

have been practised, the practitioner should rest either in *Savasana* or by just lying on the back with normal breathing. This rest should be for five minutes at the end of all the three items.

Second and Third Week of Practice
During the second week they should add the following *asanas:*

Paschimottanasana (as described in Chapter II)

Bhujangasana (as described in Chapter II)

Trikonasana (as described in Chapter V).

After practising all the *asanas* and the Pranayama mentioned above, they should now rest in *Savasana* (as described in Chapter II) for ten to fifteen minutes.

Fourth Week Onward
During the fourth week they should gradually add either all the *asanas* given below or they should choose and practise only those which they can perform comfortably:

Sarvangasana (as described in Chapter IV)

Matsyasana (as described in Chapter IV)

Dhanurasana (as described in Chapter III)

Halasana (as described below).

HALASANA
This *asana* is one of the best *asanas* of the Hatha Yoga system. It has some unique qualities and excellent benefits. Due to these, it occupies a very prominent place in the list of *asanas*. This *asana* can be performed in two ways. Though

one form is easier than the other; both have almost the same effects and rewards. Since it is a valuable *asana,* the methodological process of both forms is described and explained separartely. Let me present the easier one first.

Form 1:
Position of Readiness: Lie flat on the back. Stretch out the whole body. Make yourself quite straight. Bring the heels and toes together. Put the palms on the floor and keep them quite close to the body on both sides. Make your neck and head straight. You should be as in the readiness position of *Uttanpada Asana.* You are now ready for the actual performance.

Actual Performance: First, stretch out the legs and make them tight. Let the toes be also stretched out. Now inhale and simultaneously raise both legs upward, till they come to a vertical position. Synchronize inhaling and lifting of the legs so that you have inhaled completely when your legs have been raised. Keep both palms on the floor. Second, when you have reached the vertical point, start exhaling and simultaneously start lowering the legs towards the head area. Try to touch the floor in front of the head, Go only as far as is possible for you. Stay at the point where you can and stabilize yourself there. After the exhaling is over, keep breathing normally till the whole posture is completed. You should now be as shown in

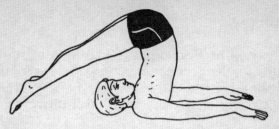

Fig. 44 *Easy Form of Halaasana.*

Fig. 44. Remain in this position for about eight to ten seconds. You are now in the Plough Pose.

Note: As long as you are in this second phase, keep the legs quite tight. Do not bend the legs. Keep the toes stretched and pointing or touching the ground. Keep both palms on the floor and the arms and hands straight and quite firm.

Third, after remaining in the second phase for about ten seconds, start returning the back to the floor. Control this returning phase. Let the back roll down on the floor, inch by inch. It is very important that you return, gradually slowly and smoothly. Keep the legs and toes quite tight all along during the returning phase. When the heels touch the ground, let the whole body relax. You have completed one round of the famous Plough posture. Now relax for six to eight seconds. Then try some more rounds in the same manner as the first one.

Daily practice Begin with two rounds. Develop it to a maximum of four rounds. A regular practice of two or three rounds would be quite satisfactory.

Form 2:

Position of Readiness: The position of readiness for this Second Form is the same as for the Form 1. Therefore, make yourself ready according to the directions given there.

Actual Performance: First, inhale and raise both hands up parallel to one another. Bring the hands in front of the head and put the back of the palms on the floor, still parallel to each other. You should synchronize your inhaling and lifting of the hands in such a way that up to the time the hands have touched the floor you have continued inhaling. When the hands touch the floor, exhale.

Second, soon after this exhaling is over, start inhaling and at the same time start lifting both legs up. Now, while inhaling, bring both legs up to a vertical position.

When the legs have reached the vertical point, start exhaling and at the same time start lowering the legs towards the floor in front of the head, and above the fingers. Now put your toes on the floor. If you cannot touch the floor with the toes, go only as far down as is possible for you. After this last exhaling is over, keep breathing normal. Do not hold the breath. Make efforts to breathe normally.

At this point, pay attention to a few things: Your legs should remain quite tense. The toes should be stretched out and on the floor or nearer to the floor side. Do not slacken or bend the knees. Try to keep the arms, hands and palms parallel to one another. With these requirements fulfilled, you are in a perfect Plough Posture as shown in Fig. 45. Stay in this position for about ten seconds.

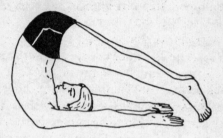

Fig. 45 *Halasana.*

Third, after being in the Plough Pose for about ten seconds, return gradually according to the following method. This returning process has the same importance as making the whole posture. Therefore pay all the attention for a smooth, slow and controlled return. Let the shoulders roll back first, then the flanks, then the small of the back, then the hip and lastly, the thighs, the legs and the heels in that order. Try to roll back inch by inch.

While returning, keep the hands on the floor, where they are. Withdraw only the legs. Roll back the whole body and let the heels fall on the floor. When the heels have touched the floor, lift both hands up and return them whilst parallel to the floor. Now put the palms on the floor. You have completed one round of the best form of the Plough Posture. Now relax. Let the

whole body relax for about six to eight seconds.
Then make a few more rounds in the same order
as the first one.

Daily practice Make one round on the first day.
Gradually go to four rounds in a few days. Four
rounds are the maximum.

Benefits: The Plough Posture has some special
values. According to Tantra Yoga, it is the
unique *asana* for gaining sexual powers. It
invigorates, energizes and nourishes all the
sexual glands and brings power, strength and
vitality to all of them. Further, it has curative
and corrective values for any weakened condition of the sex-glands. Due to these values, it
has a medicinal effect in case of impotency,
frigidity and lack of sexual power.

There are several other excellent benefits of
this *asana*. It exercises every inch of the backbone. The whole spinal cord is normalized and
soothed. Thus, so far as the flexibility of the
spine is concerned, it surpasses all other *asanas*
in effect.

The Plough Posture has an excellent effect on
correcting extra weight. It reduces excess
weight without weakening the body. It makes
the body proportionate by reducing the waist-
line, by toning up the digestive system, by
taking off fat, and by activating the whole nerve
system.

It has a very good effect on the facial area
also. Since there is speedy circulation of the
blood and since there is centralization of the

same in the upper regions, the Plough Posture nourishes the whole area and thereby increases and restores the youthful look of the face, as well as energy.

After practising the above-mentioned *asanas* the student should rest for ten to fifteen minutes in *Shavasana*. When the practice of *pranayama* and *asanas* have been regularized for about a month, they should add the practice of concentration as described below:

CONCENTRATION

Concentration is the primary step of Raja Yoga. Its next advanced stage is meditation. Before describing the method of practising concentration let me mention briefly what it is and what it does.

Concentration means consciously keeping the mind on one thing. By acquiring this power, the individual becomes master of his own mind and controls its fluctuations. His mind is not allowed the freedom to fly out and attach itself to countless issues, events, thoughts and objects. The involvement of the mind becomes selective and for some desirable purpose. Meaningless and worthless attachment is cut out. When this power of concentration is achieved through proper training, it has a great curative effect over the condition of mental sickness. This curative effect of concentration can be understood better when the nature of mind and also the mind-body relationship are explained.

Mind, by its nature, always tries to associate

itself with some issues, events, objects or
thoughts. Its involvement is with only one thing
at a time, though the duration may be for a
shorter or longer period. To what it will attach
itself is unpredictable.

This associative nature of the mind creates
one specific condition in the body, which must
be understood. As in the nature of the objects,
issues or events with which the mind attaches
itself, so it generates a likewise reaction in the
body. In other words, the nature of the reaction
is the same as is the nature of the object of
involvement. Accordingly, when the mind
attaches with something which by its nature
could arouse anger in the individual then it will
generate in his body all those conditions and
changes which anger does arouse by its very
nature. The uncalled for attachment of the
mind, by its nature, would arouse uncalled for
reactions in his bodily system resulting in times
in tension, excitement and temper and at others,
into pleasure and thrill. It is strongly held in
yoga that unless distraction of the mind is
controlled and its energy is properly channelled
towards the desired purpose, nothing worth
naming can be accomplished by the individual.
This ability to control the mind and to channel
it in the chosen direction is achieved through the
training in concentration. For practising concentration, you have to make certain preparation as described below:

Arranging the Object: Place a vase with a flower
on some piece of household furniture so that the

top of the flower is straight in front of your eyes
in the sitting position. You can put either a
bunch of flowers or a single big one in the vase.
The flower can be natural or artificial. Keep the
flower at a distance of about five feet.

Method of Practising Concentration. When the
flowers are arranged properly, be seated in an
easy pose as shown in Fig. 46. For making this
easy pose, you have to bend the knees and put
the body weight on the floor. After being in easy
pose first, bring the left hand on the lap and put
the right hand on the palm of the left hand. This
will make your right palm upwards on the top of
the left palm.

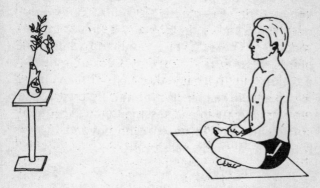

Fig. 46 *Practice of Concentration.*

Then make the body straight. Your head,
neck and the spine should be in one line and
straight upward. After the body has been
straightened up, do not tighten it. Rather, let the
body be relaxed while keeping it firm in a
straight-up position. Breathe normally. You are

now in *Sukhasana* (easy pose) as shown in Fig. 46 and ready to begin the practice of *dharana* (concentration), the first step of controlling the fluctuation of the mind. Follow the steps suggested below:

Look at the flower petals. Keep looking for about ten seconds. In case you feel any pain in the eyes, look for a shorter time. But try not to blink the eyes. When you have looked at the flower for ten seconds, close your eyes gently and try to see the shape of the flower in your mind. Keep your eyes closed for about ten seconds, while you are trying to recall the image and shape of the flower in your mind. After keeping the eyes closed for ten seconds only, open them and again look at the flower for ten seconds. Repeat this process up to five times in one session during the first week. Gradually develop it up to ten and then up to fifteen times, which should remain as the limit. If you practise ten rounds only in one session that will be quite sufficient. But, in no case go beyond fifteen rounds in a single session.

When the practice is over, keep sitting still. Now loosen the body and sit in a relaxed way for two minutes. When you have done this, your practice in concentration is complete and over.

Some Suggestions: It is suggested that after practising with a single flower for about a month, if you like you could add more flowers in the vase, though this is not necessary.

It is also suggested that after two months of practice with flowers, you could change the object. You could then practise with some photo, statue or painting of your own liking. The only consideration which you should have is about the size, colour and kind. They should be of medium size, and of soothing, pleasing but not the type likely to stir emotions.

A Word of Warning

As in any other science, the rules of Raja Yoga should also be cautiously followed in order to avoid undesirable consequences. Thus, the following warnings:

The first warning is about the limitation of time. The total time devoted to this practice of concentration should not exceed more than ten to fifteen minutes. Unless the teacher is personally guiding the practice, always keep the whole practice of concentration within the limit of ten to fifteen minutes only within a period of twenty-four hours.

The imposed limitation is necessary for some good reasons. One is that some might be fascinated by the peculiar images flashing up before their inner eye while being in the process of practice. This fascination, unless checked, might mislead one into misusing his time. Second, if anyone keeps practising for getting thrills and fascinations, then, he is not only diverting himself from the desired goal, but also taking himself to some unknown consequence which might ill-affect his actions, thoughts, performances and behaviour. A limit of time, therefore, will always keep one within the safe side of the practice where no undesirable consequence would ever be felt and known.

Testing Concentration

Whether you have gained concentration or not, you can test it yourself, according to the following guidelines. While practising, when you do not see anything through the inner eye, you have not gained concentration. While practising, when you see some other objects through your inner eye but not the one placed before your outer eyes, you are improving but still have not gained concentration. But while practising, when you see the shape of the actual object through the inner eye even for a second, you have gained concentration. When the object remains before the inner eye, in any form and shape, for up to five seconds, you have gained good concentration. When you can hold the same shape or image for up to ten seconds, you have gained a very high level of concentration. And when you have gained concentration, your mental sickness or disorders are already starting to improve.

8.

Heart Ailments and High Blood Pressure

Millions of people in the world suffer from the diseases of the heart and blood vessels, which are called 'cardiovascular diseases'. It has already become the number one killer disease in the developed countries, like the U.S.A. and Western Europe. It is also on a frightening increase in the developing countries. According to the American Medical Associaton, more than fifty per cent of all the deaths in the United States every year are caused by cardiovascular diseases and it is now called the disease of the twentieth century.

Therefore, it appears very important to know what these cardiovascular disease are; what are their causing factors; and how these diseases can be controlled, and prevented through the Therapeutic Yoga system. Since these diseases are related to the heart and the blood vessels, some basic understanding of these organs appears essential.

The heart is a tough muscular pump whose constant function is to eject blood to the arterial system at an average rate of 70 to 75 times per minute. The heart keeps the blood circulation going by receiving it in its chambers from every part of the body through the veinous system, and then by pumping it out to all parts of the body through the arteries. It is a complicated mechanism which breaks down at times in many individuals.

When any part of the circulatory system does not receive the needed blood supply, it gets damaged. This damage could be in the heart itself or in any other parts, such as, the lungs, the kidneys, the brain and other organs. That is the start of heart trouble.

The diseases associated with cardiovascular system, which can be treated through Therapeutic Yoga, are the following: atherosclerosis(hardening of the arteries), coronary thrombosis(sudden blocking of the arteries of the heart), and degenerative heart diseases, and hypertensive diseases. Let me describe briefly what these diseases are:

Atherosclerosis
The inner walls of the arteries get thickened due to gradual deposits of fatty material. These gradual deposits take the form of layers in the inner walls of the arteries and, as a result, there is hindrance to the flow of blood. Consequently, blood clotting occurs in the roughened areas and the blood circulation gets blocked.

Coronary Thrombosis
There is a *sudden blocking* of one of the arteries

or its branches and then the supply of blood to the heart is affected partially or wholly. The sudden blocking takes place due to the deposit of a clot on an already narrow artery. Due to the lack of blood supply, a heart attack may take place with pain in the chest and arms and there may be perspiration.

Degenerative Heart Disease
It occurs due to gradual decay of the blood vessels. It is thought that excessive smoking in any form causes degeneration of the blood vessels. The degenerative disease generally occurs among the middle-aged and the elderly persons. In this case, though the heart muscle continues to work, it does not possess enough strength to maintain the required healthy function.

Hypertensive Heart Disease
It occurs due to constant presence of high blood pressure in an individual. When the blood pressure continues to remain very high, it overstrains the heart muscle and also the whole of the circulatory system. This overstraining causes wear and tear on the tissues, leads to the hardening of the blood vessels, and diminishes the supply of blood to the heart and brain. Sometimes the supply of blood to the brain gets so diminished that paralysis of one or both sides of the body occurs.

It is now commonly accepted that a major cause of cardiovascular ailments is due to psychosomatic factors. The illness resulting from strain and stress is now known as psychosomatic (the word being comprised of two Greek words, *psyche* and *soma*, which mean mind and body).

The most common strain and stress are due to nervousness, which arises because of fear, anxiety, apprehension, tension and restlessness, anger, jealousy, frustration, depression and various such other feelings.

It is held in yoga that the mind controls, governs and activates the body. The body in this sense becomes a tool of the mind. What happens is that the mind-straining factors begin to also strain the bodily systems. Most of the diseases of our time, such as the heart ailments, hypertension, asthma, and various others are mostly related to these mental strains and stresses which are called in medical term 'psychosomatic factors'.

Since this chapter covers heart ailments and high blood pressure, it would be proper to describe the latter in brief before recommending their Yogic treatment.

High Blood Pressure

In a normal and healthy person the blood pressure remains 120 systolic and 80 diastolic. But when there are abnormalities in the arteries or in the circulatory system, the systolic pressure rises very high and at times, diastolic also rises.

The rise in the pressure is caused by the narrowness in the arteries, the heart has to work harder to push the blood through them and as a result of which there is high blood pressure, in medical terms this is called 'hypertension'.

Though it is normal for the blood pressure to rise high during excitement and at certain emotional moments, it usually goes down shortly. Such rises do not have any harmful effect. But when blood pressure continues to remain excessively high it causes various disorders, such as, lack of strength, tiredness, headache, and at times, difficulty in breathing, bad temper, visionary troubles, and coldness in the hands and feet.

It is now a medically established fact that hypertension may at times be due to psychosomatic factors. It could also be due to advancing age and thereby due to degenerative factors (already discussed earlier). In the following pages, the process of treatment for hypertension as well as for other heart ailments is now described:

Yogic Process of Treatment

It does not need to be emphasized that therapeutic yoga is not a treatment for an emergency case of heart attack or severe hypertension. Therapeutic yoga should only be practised when the individual concerned is not affected by an emergency type of condition.

In our treatment at the Indian Institute of Yoga, Patna, we have found that the patients of heart ailments have regained their normal health within two to three months of yoga practice. Further, once the restoration of health has been achieved, the patients remain in good health without any complaint. Likewise, in cases of high blood pressure, we have found that normalization of the circulatory system occurs within one to two months when the patient has been co-operative in following our instructions.

It is significant to mention that the yoga system of treatment is the same for heart ailments as for hypertension. The treatment comprises three steps: *(i)* observance to certain principles and advice, *(ii)* eating a proper diet, and *(iii)* practising yoga on selected basis. Let me explain first some important principles and advice.

Principles and Advice: They should stop smoking cigarettes and the use of tobacoo in any form, and should give up taking tea and coffee. Alcoholic drinks should be discontinued. Intake of butter, cream, eggs, meat, excessive fat containing food items should be stopped.

Hot spices, pickles, chutney, red chilli, and excessive use of salt should be excluded from the eating items. Avoid over-eating at all times. Rest and relaxation is absolutely vital.

For a detailed understanding about diet, bathing, cleaning, and other yogic principles, the users of this section are advised to read thoroughly the first chapter of this book. Some important advice which is not covered in the first chapter, is mentioned below:

One major piece of advice is to be relaxed and keep yourself free from anxiety, nervousness, tension and restlessness. Though it is not easy for every individual to be relaxed in every condition and situation, it can be done with proper understanding about the self, society and the nature. These aspects are discussed in Chapter VII of this book and you are advised to read it properly for developing self-power for overcoming these tension-creating problems. With these suggestions, the diet-chart for the heart ailments patients is now described.

DIET CHART

Breakfast (7 to 9 a.m.)
(i) Any fruit juice – One cup or sweet orange
(ii) Any fresh fruit – One or as desired (except mangoes and lichi)
(iii) Germinated gram – 1/4 cup
(iv) Wheat bread or toast – as desired
(v) Skimmed milk (if desired) – One cup
Lunch and Dinner (12 noon to 2 p.m.: 6 – 8 p.m.)
(i) Salad (a mixture of tomato, cucumber, radish, lettuce, carrot, etc., with very little salt and lemon juice or with french dressing or plain) – one cup
(ii) Vegetable soup – one cup
(iii) Wheat bread – as desired
(iv) Pulse (e.g. green pea) – as desired
(v) (Leafy vegetables of any kind) – as desired
(vi) Green vegetables (of any kind) – as desired
Fish (for non-vegetarians) – 2 moderate pieces

Afternoon snack (3 to 5 p.m.)
(i) Fresh fruit of any type – as desired
(ii) Salted biscuits – as desired
The important points to be kept in mind are that
the major part of every day diet should be of
salad, fresh fruits and green vegetables. Dishes
should be cooked in vegetable oils using little or
no spices.

Yoga Practice
The patients of heart ailments and hypertension
should practise yoga, in phases, according to
the guidelines given below:

First Phase: It should last for three weeks. In
this phase, only *Savasana* needs to be practised.
A detailed description about the method of
practising *Savasava* is given in Chapter II. The
patient should first read and develop a proper
understanding about the process of *Savasana*
before actually practising it. One important
piece of advice is, practise it slowly. Do it
thoroughly and with patience.

Daily Practice: *Savasana* should be practised
twice or thrice daily. At one stretch, it should
be performed for about thirty to forty minutes.
The most suitable times for practising it, are in
the morning (before breakfast), in the afternoon
(2 hours after lunch), and in the evening. The
main consideration is that the stomach should
be empty and not heavy with food.
. Those suffering from high blood pressure

should get themselves examined to find out their condition after practising *Savasana* for three weeks. By this time, the blood pressure should be normalized. When the blood pressure becomes normal, they should add the *asanas* of the second and the third phase described below. But in case the blood pressure remains more than 150 systolic, they should keep practising only *Savasana*, till normalization occurs.

Benefits: Though the benefits of *Savasana* are already mentioned in Chapter II, a few words need to be added here. Our experience shows that a regular and proper practice of *Savasana* for about two to three weeks brings a remarkable effect on the patients of heart ailments and of high blood pressure. It corrects the disorders of the circulatory system by relaxing the nerves and the internal organs. Because of this normalizing and relaxing effect on the arteries, high blood pressure is reduced and gradually it is corrected.

Second Phase (Fourth and Fifth Weeks): Before practising yoga of this phase, the practiser must read the Essentials of Yoga Practice as described in Chapter I with special attention to the requirements of rest. After practising *Savasana* twice or thrice daily during the first phase, the following *asanas* should be added. Now yoga practice should be performed in the order listed below:

(i) *Pawanmuktasana*: (In lying position): It is comprehensively described in Chapter II. Practise it without straining yourself. Do only as much as you can comfortably. Make four to six rounds daily.

(ii) Uttanpadasana: (with only one leg at a time) – It is fully described in Chapter II. In the beginning, hold the leg up for only a few seconds. Gradually increase the time to four, then to six seconds. Daily practice should be only six rounds (three rounds with each leg).

(iii) Savasana: When other *asanas* are practised *Savasana* should be done at the end. Method of practising *Savasana* remains the same as during the first phase. Duration of *Savasana* when done after yoga practice, may be reduced if desired. A practice of fifteen to thirty minutes should be sufficient.

During this second phase, *Savasana* should be practised singly also, at least one more time during a period of twenty-four hours.

Third Phase (Sixth Week Onwards): During this phase and onward, the daily practice of yoga should be in the following order:

(i) Pranayama (with Rechaka and Puraka) – Its method of practice is illustrated and described in Chapter II. Practise according to the directions given therein.

(ii) Surya Namaskar asana – As described in Chapter III.

(iii) Santulanasana – As described in Chapter V.

(iv) Pawanmuktasana – As done earlier.

(v) Uttanpadasana – As done earlier.

(vi) Savasana – As done earlier.

Other recommended books:

ACUPRESSURE TECHNIQUES
FOR THE SELF-TREATMENT OF MINOR AILMENTS

Dr. Hans Ewald. *Illustrated.* Acupressure was developed from the Chinese healing system of acupuncture. It makes use of the same points and meridians (paths), but thumbs and forefingers are used instead of needles. Its prime use is in alleviating and healing nervous diseases, with particular reference to nervous exhaustion, anxiety states, heart and circulatory disturbances, impotence, frigidity, insomnia, headaches, and skin complaints. The technique is explained lucidly in this excellent handbook. Pictures and supplementary drawings indicate the exact location of the points, which should be activated in a clockwise direction for between one and five minutes. Beneficial reaction is quick and lasts for some time.

CHINESE MICRO-MASSAGE
Acupuncture Without Needles

J. Lavier. *Illustrated.* Bridging the gap between classical massage and acu-puncture micro-massage activates tiny points below the skin—either by hand or special instruments—and this action produces amazingly therapeutic results! It is an ideal therapy for squeamish patients or children who are afraid of having their flesh punctured, even minutely, by acupuncture needles. Although the *mechanical* action of micro-massage is feeble compared to massage proper, its uniquely *energizing* effect may be likened to the stimulation electrologists impart to muscles by the application of small electrodes. *Includes:* General technique; How to use the massage-points; Treatment of rheumatism.

PRESS POINT THERAPY

Gerard J. Bendix. *Illustrated.* Help yourself (and others) banish the pain of backache, headache, sinus, haemorrhoids, etc., by manipulating press points in the feet. These mark nerve-like connecting pathways leading to all parts of the body and are connector points to vital glands, nerves and organs! Manipulation of these points can also delay the signs and effects of ageing— prevent oncoming or existing poor states of health—discover potential health complications almost before they occur—relieve nervous tension—and provide a quick energizer. You will be amazed how quickly you will locate the press points in your own—or somebody else's—feet. As you start feeling the bene-ficial effects, Press Point Therapy grows on you. The results speak for them-selves!

REFLEXOLOGY
THE TECHNIQUES OF FOOT MASSAGE
FOR HEALTH AND FITNESS

Anna Kaye and Don Matchan. *Illustrated.* Explains techniques of foot mas-sage, the natural way of stimulating internal organs for restoring body functions to normal. This is an ancient art, used by the Chinese for more than 5,000 years. It is practised primarily on the feet because *in the feet are mirrored all organs of the body*. Treatment details given for allergies, arthritis, asthma. colds, constipa-tion, diabetes, digestive troubles, emphysema, headache, high blood-pressure, muscle cramps, varicose veins, weight problems, hot flushes, etc. Includes chart showing locations of the reflexes and a chapter on American Indian massage.

INTRODUCTION TO HATHA YOGA
THE WAY TO HEALTH, HAPPINESS AND FULFILMENT

Margaret Perkins. *Illustrated.* Shows how simple yoga exercises can help you to relax and enjoy health, happiness and fulfilment. Look and feel more attractive with a daily yoga practice! It differs from physical culture in that the emphasis is not on muscle-building but rather on controlling and using our bodies correctly. There is no emphasis on strength or speed and it is not competitive. The asanas (poses) and exercises are largely aimed at toning up the nervous system. Chapters on yoga breathing, food and diet, concentration and positive thinking.

PRACTICAL YOGA

Harvey Day The type of Yoga contained in this book is known as Hatha Yoga and is chiefly concerned with development of the physical body. But Yoga will not create a muscle-bound 'Mr Universe'; it is designed to make limbs and organs healthy. It is not meant primarily for the young (who can perform most of the postures with comparative ease), but for the middle-aged; those who suffer from obesity or arthritis; those whose breathing may be laboured and wheezy. Yoga breathing, combined with the exercises, should produce impressive benefits for the regular practitioner. He or she can acquire an easy carriage, lissom body, a magical sense of physical well-being and a deep-seated feeling of serenity.

CHINESE YOGA
INTERNAL EXERCISES FOR HEALTH AND SERENITY OF BODY AND MIND

Stephen T. Chang. *Illustrated.* Internal exercises, devised by Taoist sages over 6,000 years ago, for relieving over 30 common ailments, including headaches, colds, constipation, blood pressure, female problems, and insomnia. The exercises are modelled on the deer, crane, and turtle, animals noted for their longevity. They conserve and build up body energy—unlike external exercises, which expend energy without replacing it. They are designed to energize the entire body, balance the energy level, promote a more effective functioning of internal organs.

AROMA-THERAPY
THE USE OF PLANT ESSENCES IN HEALING

Raymond Lautié D.Sc. Describes a selection of essential oils expressed from herbs and plants and their external and internal applications for a host of ailments, including arthritis, colds, flu, liver ailments, rheumatism, sleeplessness and ulcers. Essential oils respect living tissues and are generally less toxic than laboratory drugs. Here they are examined in alphabetical order and in each case their main therapeutic qualities are indicated. Oils dealt with include arnica, basil, coriander, elecampane, eucalyptus, fennel, garlic, ledum (wild rosemary), marjoram, mugwort, orange (Seville), pine (Scots), sage, sandalwood, thyme and valerian. A therapeutic, ancient art revived!

DEFEATING DEPRESSION

A GUIDE FOR DEPRESSED PEOPLE AND THEIR FAMILIES

C. A. H. Watts O.B.E., M.D. Depression is a treatable illness! Here is a doctor's concise guide to the various types of depression and to therapies that can bring help, hope and comfort to sufferers. This sympathetic and informative book has been specially written for all those to whom depression has become a fact of life. *Contents include:* What is mental depression? Reactive and symptomatic depression; Causes of depression; The role of the psychiatrist; Other sources of help; The Church and the Samaritans; Talking through the problem; Low mood syndromes and vitamin deficiencies; The dangers of tranquillizers.

LINDA CLARK'S HANDBOOK OF NATURAL REMEDIES

FOR COMMON AILMENTS

Linda Clark. Shows how common ailments, including allergies, arthritis, constipation, high blood-pressure and heart trouble, may be treated naturally by nutrition, herbs, homoeopathy, osteopathy, and other methods. Nature works through all systems of healing and we should take advantage of every source, however unorthodox. Colour therapy, chiropractic, contact therapy and acupressure are other means of treating disease. In this book you will almost certainly find an efficacious new healing approach to whatever ails *you*!

RELIEF FROM ARTHRITIS

A SAFE AND EFFECTIVE TREATMENT FROM THE OCEAN

John E. Croft, F.C.S. 60% of rheumatoid arthritis and 30-50% of osteoarthritis sufferers tested with extract from New Zealand green-lipped mussels were relieved of symptoms! (Some were chronic cases). This book explains why. Green-lipped mussels are cultivated on marine farms and the therapeutic substance extracted is rich in amino acids and minerals, resulting in a treatment that is both safe and effective and which gives hope for freedom from pain and for the restoration of mobility to many sufferers from arthritis. Extract now available in Britain from health food stores and chemists.

HEALING WITH RADIONICS

THE SCIENCE OF HEALING ENERGY

E. Baerlein & A. L. G. Dower. *Illustrated.* Radionic practitioners believe that all matter radiates its own wavelength and that living organisms emit electromagnetic wave radiations which depend on psycho-physical health for their intensity and frequency. This book traces the growth of radionic therapy and describes diagnostic instruments and methods of treating illness in humans and animals. *Contents include:* The theory of radionics; Radionic instruments; Ruth Drown, a major figure in radionics; The Delawarr camera; The 'magnetogeometric potency simulator'; Training in radionics; The Pendulum; Radionic analysis—subtle anatomy; Human and animal case histories; Radionics in agriculture.

VITAMIN E: The Vitality Vitamin
WHAT IT IS AND WHY YOU NEED IT

Dr Leonard Mervyn. 'The wonder worker' vitamin E is an invaluable aid in the treatment of such disorders as thrombosis, heart disease, and skin complaints. It can also prevent kidney disease, high blood-pressure, blindness and gangrene in diabetics. In this book Dr Mervyn explains how to obtain the optimum intake of vitamin E from dietary and supplementary sources. *Includes:* Vitamin E, its discovery, properties and dietary requirements; Natural sources of vitamin E; Deficiencies and how to overcome them; What vitamin E does in the body; Some conditions that have been helped by vitamin E.

ISOMETRICS
THE SHORT STEP TO FITNESS

James Hewitt. *Illustrated.* Explains static muscle contractions, produced by exerting steady pressure in held positions without limb movement. You only need the space you stand in, a programme takes just a few minutes, but the result can be improved health and appearance—even for the bed-bound and disabled, who are here provided with isometrics to do in bed. *Includes:* General rules for practice; Programme for men; Programme for women; Programme for muscle power; Programme of sitting exercises; Programme of exercises in bed; Exercises with a partner; Isometrics for the face; Guide to contracting muscle groups.

OSTEOPATHY
Head-to-Toe Health Through Manipulation

Leon Chaitow N.D., D.O. *Illustrated.* Incorrect posture constitutes a health hazard, while few women realize that wearing high heels can produce lordosis (tilting forward of the pelvis). Here a practising osteopath explains the correct way to walk, sit and sleep; provides simple exercises to improve abdominal tone, correct stooped shoulders and flat chests; demonstrates a method of relaxation for releasing physical tensions. The author further reveals an interesting development known as 'cranial osteopathy'. This entails manipulation of the skull to correct adverse effects of head injuries caused by blows, tooth extraction, or even the warping of pliable skull bones at birth.

EVERYBODY'S GUIDE TO NATURE CURE

The most comprehensive treatise on Nature Cure that has ever been published containing 486 pages of unrivalled health knowledge. Part 1 deals with Nature Cure in Theory and Outline. Part 2 describes fully the self-treatment of Child Ailments, Diseases of the Skin and Scalp; Joints and Rheumatic Affections; The Blood, Blood-Vessels and Circulatory System; Nerves and Nervous System; Eyes; Ears, Nose. Mouth and Throat; Stomach and Intestines; Heart Lungs, Bronchial Tubes, and Larynx; Liver, Gall-Bladder, Kidneys, Bladder and Pancreas; Male and Female Sex Organs. Deals with Fevers and Influenza and contains General Treatments, Diets, First-Aid etc.—and is comprehensively indexed for easy reference.